NATUR GROW OWN HEALTH GARDEN

N H Hawes

Hammersmith Health Books
London, UK

First published in 2017 by Hammersmith Health Books – an imprint of
Hammersmith Books Limited
4/4A Bloomsbury Square, London WC1A 2RP
www.hammersmithbooks.co.uk

© 2017 N H Hawes

All rights reserved. No part of this publication may be reproduced, stored in
any retrieval system or transmitted in any form or by any means, electronic,
mechanical, photocopying, recording or otherwise, without the prior permission
of the publisher and the copyright holder.

Note: No book can replace the diagnostic expertise and medical advice
of a trusted physician. Please be certain to consult your doctor before making any
decisions that affect your health or extreme changes to your diet, particularly if
you suffer from any medical condition or have any symptom that may require
treatment. Whilst the advice and information in this book are believed to be true
and accurate at the date of going to press, neither the author nor the publisher
can accept any legal responsibility or liability for any errors or omissions that
may have been made.

British Library Cataloguing in Publication Data: A CIP record of this book is
available from the British Library.

ISBN (print edition): 978-1-78161-081-7
ISBN (ebook): 978-1-78161-082-4

Commissioning editor: Georgina Bentliff
Cover design by: Julie Bennett, Bespoke Publishing Ltd
Typeset by: Julie Bennett, Bespoke Publishing Ltd
Production: Helen Whitehorn, Path Projects Ltd
Printed and bound by: TJ International Ltd

Contents

	About Nature Cures	4
1.	Introduction	5
2.	Planning your organic health garden	6
3.	Plants that do not mind partial shade	8
4.	Why crop rotation is important	9
5.	Natural pest control	11
6.	What crops to grow health-wise	20
7.	Feeding your health-garden plants	93
8.	Growing food crops in pots indoors	98
9.	Growing sprouts on your windowsill	99
10.	Plants that are poisonous to pets and young children	103
	Index	110
	About the author	112

About Nature Cures

This pocketbook is a guide to natural ways to treat health issues. The information is drawn from my website www.naturecures.co.uk and my comprehensive book *Nature Cures: The A to Z of Ailments and Natural Foods*, available from www.hammersmithbooks.co.uk. For more detail about the nutrients and foods listed in this pocketbook, please do refer to these sources.

In both this book and my comprehensive works the sources of the information I've used are too numerous to list without at least doubling the size; if there is any fact or recommendation that is of concern, please do contact me via www.naturecures.co.uk.

This pocketbook represents a compilation of years of research but is no substitute for visiting a qualified health practitioner so please do consult such, especially your doctor with regard to any prescription medications, before making signficant changes to your diet, lifestyle or health regime.

Other books in this series
Recovery from Injury, Surgery and Infection
Nature's Colour Codes
Let Roots Be Your Medicine
Air-purifying Houseplants

Introduction

The best way to ensure that you, your family and friends consume only organic, untainted and nutrient-rich foods is to grow your own herbs, fruits and vegetables. This can be done in the smallest of plots or even on a balcony, roof garden or windowsill with a raised box or pots and other types of planters. Outside, fences, railings and walls can be utilised with canvas pocket planters, mounted boxes and hanging baskets, or be inventive and hang up old bottles and containers with holes pierced or drilled in the bottom.

A very good way to grow food crops, especially for those less able, is to have raised beds built. These can easily be made from old pallets and can be two or three feet high to provide an easily accessed planter even for those who are wheelchair bound. If these beds are surrounded with gravel and sharp sand paths it will also deter garden pests like slugs and snails. Protect the wood with natural linseed oil, which has excellent preservative properties and is water resistance and harmless to wildlife and humans.

Planning your organic health garden

Growing plants from seeds is very easy and rewarding. Always purchase organic seeds in the first place; these may be slightly more expensive but, after the first season's harvest, seeds can be collected from home-grown plants and are therefore forever free thereafter.

When planning a garden, it is important to add as many native plants as possible to support the local wildlife and beneficial insects, like bees, that will pollinate the herbs, fruits and vegetables you want to grow. Filling your outside space with alien species simply for their looks or colour is a sorry waste of valuable space that could feed native flora and fauna as well as your family, friends and neighbours.

The easiest edible plants to begin growing are:

- bell peppers
- chilli peppers
- broad and runner beans
- carrots
- herbs
- peas
- potatoes
- strawberries
- sunflowers
- tomatoes
- turnips

These can all be grown in pots or other containers if space is restricted. In small spaces, use a large container or pot with a cane tee-pee to grow beans and peas, along with sweet peas to help attract pollinating insects. Potatoes are a good first crop, when growing directly in the ground, as they will break up the soil and add nutrients that future vegetables will require.

What many consider as weeds are often very powerful medicinal plants; these include nettles and dandelions - teas made from these are very beneficial for the body plus they are attractive to beneficial pollinating insects. Nettles can also be used to make your own crop-feed; do this by soaking a large bunch of them in a large covered container of water for one week, then strain off the water and keep it to feed crops once a week. This nettle water can also be used in a spray to wash off aphids.

NOTE: Some plants must be grown in containers as otherwise they spread very rapidly; examples include bamboo, borage, dandelions, mint, nettles and peppermint.

Plants that do not mind partial shade

In a small garden or balcony, there is often a lack of full sun throughout the day and many believe that they cannot grow crops in these circumstances. However, as long as there are a few hours of sunshine on them during some part of the day, the following plants will grow quite happily in partial shade, although they will also thrive in full sun.

- Beans
- Beetroot
- Broccoli
- Brussel sprouts
- Burdock
- Cauliflower
- Chamomile
- Cress
- Echinacea
- Endive
- Ginger
- Kale
- Lettuce
- Milk thistle
- Mustard
- Oregano
- Peas
- Rocket
- Spinach
- Turnip

Why crop rotation is important

Annual crop rotation is used to control pests and diseases that can become established in the soil over time because plants within the same taxonomic family tend to have similar pests and pathogens. Changing crops annually also reduces the chance of nutrient deficiencies developing in the soil and food crops with large leaves and dense foliage will suppress weeds for the crops that are planted in that place next time.

Certain annual crops, such as cucurbits (courgettes, cucumbers, marrow, pumpkins and squashes), salads (endive, lettuce and chicory) and sweetcorn and sweet potatoes can be grown anywhere but should not be grown too often in the same place.

There are three categories of plants for your crop rotation bed as follows:

1. Potatoes
2. Legumes (beans and peas), onions and other root vegetables (except turnip and swede)
3. Brassicas (which include bok choy, broccoli, Brussels sprouts, cabbage, cauliflower, Chinese cabbage, collard greens, cress, daikon, horseradish, kale, kohlrabi, mizuna,

mustard greens, radish, rapeseed, rocket, shepherd's purse, swede, turnip, wasabi, watercress).

First, divide your health garden into three sections with an extra one for the perennials, such as rhubarb and asparagus, that do not need to be rotated. Then plant your crops in each section as follows.

Year one

- Section one: Potatoes
- Section two: Legumes, onions and roots
- Section three: Brassicas

Year two

- Section one: Brassicas
- Section two: Potatoes
- Section three: Legumes, onions and roots

Year three

- Section one: Legumes, onions and roots
- Section two: Brassicas
- Section three: Potatoes

Natural garden pest control

A bird-feeding station is important to attract birds as these will consume many garden pests, such as caterpillars, slugs and snails. However, in some urban areas, bird food can also attract mice, rats and foxes, so care should be taken.

Hedgehogs will consume many garden pests that attack food crops. Leaving a pile of logs and twigs undisturbed or building a hedgehog house will help to keep hedgehogs in the garden providing there is a way for them to get into the garden in the first place.

A pond is a valuable asset as it too will encourage the wild life that can help to control pests. Frogs, dragonflies, damsel flies, newts and toads will consume many of the unwanted garden pests encountered in your health garden. To naturally reduce algae growth in a pond, add some tied up nets of barley straw for six weeks before replacing and a sprinkle of wood ash now and then can help, as can adding plenty of pond plants and water snails.

Ants, aphids, black fly, green fly and white fly

Aphids can attack a wide variety of plants depending on their species. Many will thrive upon beans, cabbage, cucumber, melons, peas, potatoes, pumpkin, squash and tomatoes. Green aphids thrive on roses, grey ones on brassicas, black ones on broad beans and white ones on box hedges.

Aphids can also transmit viruses from one plant to another, especially beans, beetroot, bok choy, cucumber, lettuce, melons, potatoes, pumpkins, squashes and Swiss chard. These viruses can mottle, yellow or curl leaves and stunt plant growth.

Ants protect aphids, as they feed on the honeydew aphids produce, so must also be removed. Control ants by trimming the lower parts of the plant so that they do not touch the ground and give ants easy access. The use of an organic aphid control pesticide, such as neem oil, will take care of the ants as well.

Natural ant repellents
- **Apple juice**: Place a cup of apple juice near to the plants where aphids are present and the ants will climb into the cup and drown in the juice.
- **Baking soda, sugar and yeast**: Sprinkle the ants' path with a mixture of these. Sugar will attract them and baking soda and yeast will eliminate them.
- **Bay leaves**: Place dried bay leaves around the plants you want to protect.

- **Chilli pepper** destroys the chemical signals that ants rely on to navigate towards food. Sprinkle on the ants' pathways.
- **Cinnamon and cloves**: can successfully deter ants if placed near to their usual routes.
- **Eucalyptus oil**: Spray the diluted oil on their usual routes and this will deter them from returning.
- **Flower of sulphur**: Pour a trail of flower-of-sulphur powder around the ants' nest.
- **Honey**: An open jar of honey will attract ants and they will become stuck inside the jar.
- **Lemons**: The scent of lemon deters ants and its acidic property masks their scent trails. Place some slices of lemon around where they reside and spray lemon juice on their usual trails.
- **Peppermint**: Ants hate the strong aroma which also disrupts their smelling capabilities so they cannot detect food sources. Use peppermint oil and dried leaves around the plants where any aphids are present to deter the ants.
- **Tea tree oil**: Spray onto the ants' pathways to deter them.
- **Vinegar** removes the trails ants leave to use as a pathway to their feeding places. Dilute a tablespoon of vinegar with water in a sprayer and spray on to the pathways they use near to vegetables.

Combination plants for pest control
Growing the following plants close to each other will protect against

the aphids and other bugs that can attack the vegetables mentioned. These plants can be in pots nearby or in the ground.

- **Basil**: tomatoes
- **Chives**: sunflowers and tomatoes
- **Leeks**: carrots
- **Marigolds**: tomatoes
- **Mint**: broccoli, Brussel sprouts, cabbage, carrots, cauliflower, kale and tomatoes
- **Nasturtiums**: beans, broccoli, Brussels sprouts, cabbage, cauliflower, kale and peas
- **Peppermint**: cabbage, cucumber, melons, peas, potatoes, pumpkin, squash and tomatoes
- **Spring onions**: carrots.

Beneficial insects for pest control

Attracting the following beneficial insects to the garden is a natural way to kill garden pests; for instance, one ladybird will consume 5000 aphids during its yearlong lifetime.

- Assassin bugs (*Reduviidae*)
- Big eyed bugs (*Geocoris*)
- Damsel bug (*Nabidae*)
- Damselfly (*Zygoptera*)
- Dragonfly (*Anisoptera*)
- Enscarpia wasps (*Encyrtidae*)
- Gall midge (*Aphidoletes aphidimyza*)
- Hoverfly (*Syrphidae*)
- Lacewing (*Chrysopidae*)
- Ladybird (*Coccinellidae*, ladybugs)
- Longhorn beetle (*Cerambycidae*)
- Minute pirate bug

- (*Anthocoridae*)
- Parasitic wasps (*Trichogrammatidae*)
- Praying mantis (*Mantodea*)
- Soldier beetle (*Cantharidae*, leatherwing)
- Stink bugs (*Pentatomidae*)

Nearby plantings of the following will help to attract these beneficial insects to your garden, if left to flower, as many insect predators also consume pollen.

- Borage
- Buddleia
- Caraway
- Carrots
- Celery
- Coriander
- Cow parsley
- Dandelion
- Dill
- Fennel
- Golden marguerite
- Lovage
- Mint
- Parsnips
- Parsley
- Scented stocks
- Sweet peas
- Yarrow

The planting of the following, which are attractive to aphids, are good for organic aphid control. Growing these in a separate space from fruit and vegetables will lure aphids away and will also attract the predators of aphids, such as ladybirds, which will, in turn, help to control aphids on the food crops.

- Asters
- Begonias
- Chrysanthemums
- Cosmos

- Dahlias
- Geraniums
- Hollyhocks
- Larkspur
- Roses
- Verbena
- Zinnia

Other ways to control aphids

- **Chives, garlic, leeks, onions and spring onions** will also help to deter aphids as they do not like the odour; therefore, grow them amongst the crops susceptible to attack.
- **Cucumber**: Place a few slices in a small aluminium pie tin around the garden to remain free of pests all season long. The chemicals in the cucumber react with the aluminium to give off a scent undetectable to humans but which will make most garden pests flee the area.
- **Stinging nettle tea** can be used as an aphid killer. Soak half a pound of nettles in a bucket of water for a week, before straining and using undiluted to control aphids. This is also beneficial to the plants as it will feed them.
- **Water**: A few aphids will not cause too much damage and are part of the balance of a healthy vegetable garden. Rubbing them off with the fingers or plain water in a powerful sprayer is often enough to keep them at bay.

Slugs and snails

When disposing of snails, it is pointless (as well as selfish) to simply throw them into your neighbour's garden as they have a powerful homing instinct and will return the next night.

Never use salt to kill slugs and snails as this causes them great pain for some time before they die.

- **Beer traps**: Slugs and snails are attracted to beer so a small jar half filled with beer will trap and drown them so that they can be disposed of on the compost heap or a bird table.
- **Coffee grounds**: These can be sprinkled around plants as a safe deterrent but do not use too often.
- **Copper**: Slugs and snails get electric shocks from copper so it is a useful tool to stop them getting near to your vegetables. It will not harm them but will deter them. Self-adhesive copper bands can be used around pots and planters.
- **Diatomaceous earth and sharp sand**: Diatomaceous earth comes in the form of a chalky powder and is the natural fossilised remains of diatoms, a type of hard-shelled algae. Both this powder and sharp sand make a good barrier to slugs and snails as they cannot easily cross it if it is sprinkled around vegetables or planters and raised beds.
- **Electric barrier**: Small electric ribbons which run off a nine-volt battery can be purchased and set up around vegetables. When a slug or snail comes in contact with the fence, it receives a mild static sensation that is undetectable to animals

and humans. This does not kill the slug but causes it to look elsewhere for forage.

- **Grapefruit and flower pot traps**: Place half a grapefruit skin or a flower pot upturned near to your vegetables with a small stone to raise one side. This will attract slugs and snails, which can be disposed of in the morning. The grapefruit scent attracts them so is often a better solution. A wide plank can be used in the same way as slugs and snails will use it for shelter during the day. There is no need to kill them. Simply take them to a wildlife habitat at least two miles away from your garden.
- **Lava rock**: can be used as a barrier around plantings, but should be left mostly above soil level, otherwise dirt or vegetation soon forms a bridge for slugs to cross.
- **Seaweed**: has the added benefit of adding nutrients to the soil if used as a mulch around vegetables. Pile it on three to four inches (7-10 centimetres) thick - when it dries it will shrink to just an inch (2.5 centimetres) or so deep. Seaweed is salty and slugs and snails avoid salt. Push the seaweed away from plant stems so it's not in direct contact. During hot weather, seaweed will dry out and become very rough which also deters the slugs.
- **Watering schedule**: If watering is only done in the early morning the soil dries out by the time snails and slugs become active at night. This can reduce slug and snail attacks by 80%.
- **Wood ash**: Providing the plants concerned do not prefer an acidic soil, wood ash can be used around plants to deter slugs

and snails. However, once it rains this deterrent is rendered useless and needs to be reapplied.

Spider mites

Spider mites thrive upon asparagus, beans, melons, squash and other cucurbits, peas, tomatoes and strawberries, as well as several weed species. The same methods can be used to remove them as with the aphids.

What crops to grow health-wise

Nature has kindly colour-coded foods for us and each colour denotes specific nutrients important to health. This means it is important to grow some foods of each colour to gain optimum nutrition from your health garden. Below you will find a list of the healthiest food crops that grow well in temperate climates and how they can benefit the health of you, your family, your neighbours and your friends.

A note about 'free radicals' and 'antioxidants'

Throughout the descriptions of beneficial plants below there are references to the importance of preventing 'free radical damage' with the aid of 'antioxidants'. They are therefore prefaced with the following explanation.

'Free radicals' and 'antioxidants' are terms used to explain intricate molecular processes which would take up too much space to explain fully in this pocketbook but are described in depth on the Nature Cures 'Cleanse and Detoxify' page on the naturecures.co.uk website and in the comprehensive volume *Nature Cures*.

Put simply, a free radical is a molecule that is missing an

electron. Because of this it is unstable and reactive and attacks other molecules to steal an electron in order to become stable again. But the molecule it steals the electron from then becomes a free radical and this causes a chain reaction, like a domino effect, which can lead to cell damage within the body.

Heavy metal molecules can greatly intensify this reaction, if they collide with free radicals, causing far greater damage, which may be one of the root causes of Alzheimer's and other brain degeneration diseases.

Many factors can induce free-radical formation in the environment. They cause clothes to fade, food to spoil, metal to rust, pipes to leak, plastics to deteriorate, paint to fade and peel and works of art to degrade.

In the human body, free radicals can be useful because they help important reactions to take place. They arise normally during metabolism and sometimes the immune system's white blood cells purposefully create them to neutralise bacteria and viruses. Free radicals are a natural by-product of the body when it turns food into energy and, normally, the body makes its own antioxidant enzymes to deal with them. Catalase, glutathione peroxidase and superoxide dismutase are three such enzymes and they require micronutrient cofactors such as copper, iron, manganese, selenium and zinc for their activity.

An excess of free radicals becomes a problem because they attack the body itself, damaging key cellular molecules, such as DNA (our genetic code). Cells with damaged DNA are more prone to developing cancer, and free radical damage accumulates with age.

An antioxidant is not actually a substance; it is a behaviour.

Any compound that can donate electrons to eliminate free radicals, without becoming a free radical itself, has antioxidant properties.

Some antioxidant molecules are too big to go through the gut wall so they work in the gut itself. Some antioxidants are water-soluble so can go where the fat-soluble ones cannot. Some work on the surface of cells and some work inside cells. Because different antioxidants work in different areas of the body, the key is to eat as wide a range of foods with antioxidant abilities as possible.

Compounds with antioxidant abilities

- Alpha-carotene
- Alpha-lipoic acid
- Astaxanthin
- Beta-carotene
- Beta-cryptoxanthin
- Carnitine
- Catalase
- Catechins
- Coenzyme Q10
- Flavonoids
- Glutathione
- Iridium
- Lutein and zeaxanthin
- Lycopene
- Manganese
- Melatonin
- Phenols and polyphenols
- Phytoestrogens
- Quercetin
- Resveratrol
- Selenium
- Superoxide dismutase
- Uric acid
- Vitamin A
- Vitamin C
- Vitamin E

Many of the natural foods that can be grown in your health garden contain these antioxidants and the nutrients the body requires to make its own antioxidants, as described here.

Vegetables

Home-grown organic vegetables will taste so much better than shop-bought versions and this is due to the richer concentration of nutrients which will occur when the soil is looked after well and the plants are fed naturally. Intensely farmed crops leech many minerals from the soil which are not replaced and artificial fertilisers, fungicides, herbicides and pesticides are often used to increase yield (and hence profits), which can leave toxic residues in food crops that are then ingested by humans.

Many people do not realise the exceptional nutritional value of the leaves and skins of root vegetables and throw them away. Many vegetables leaves are edible (except those from the nightshade family) and should be shredded and lightly steamed. Examples of leaves that can be consumed this way are beetroot, carrots, cauliflower, radishes, swede and turnips. Even the root tips of radishes contain valuable nutrients.

The skins of most vegetables are where most nutrients are concentrated so peeling them should be avoided. This is true of carrots, potatoes, sweet potatoes, turnips and young fresh swedes. Many root vegetables that are normally cooked, can also be grated and eaten raw if they are harvested when they are young and small. The exception to this is the potato which must always be cooked before eating.

Broccoli, cauliflower and kale leaves (and thin slices of swede or sweet potatoes) can be lightly baked then sprinkled with Himalayan pink salt crystals or unrefined sea salt to provide a more nutritious alternative to potato crisps.

NOTE: In order to absorb the fat-soluble beta carotene in vegetables they must be eaten with fat-rich foods such as cold-pressed nut, seed or other plant oils like coconut, olive or rice bran oils or fish oils or avocado.

Alfalfa *(Medicago sativa)*
Alfalfa is known as 'The father of all foods' because it contains just about everything the body needs for survival. It is easy to grow in the ground and provides a good green crop to grow in a bed that has had root vegetables grown in it previously. Then it can be dug in to overwinter and this will provide many nutrients in the soil for the next vegetable crop. Another way to grow alfalfa seeds is in a jam jar on a windowsill to provide highly nutritious salad sprouts. See Grow Sprouts on Your Windowsill below (page 100).

Artichoke *(Cynara scolymus,* globe artichoke)
The globe artichoke is a thistle vegetable of Mediterranean origin and should not be confused with the Jerusalem artichoke. They can be grown easily, even in a flower bed, and usually flower in the same year as the seeds are sown.

Artichoke contains the bitter components cynarin and sesquiterpene-lactones which inhibit cholesterol synthesis and increase its excretion in the bile, which results in cholesterol reduction in the blood. They also help to cleanse the liver and to protect against hepatitis and skin cancer. Artichoke is also a good source of silymarin, caffeic acid and ferulic acid, which help to protect the body from harmful free-radical agents.

The artichoke is additionally a rich source of vitamin B9 (folate), which acts as a co-factor for enzymes involved in the synthesis of DNA. Regular consumption of foods rich in vitamin B9 during the pre-conception period, and during early pregnancy, helps prevent neural tube defects, including spina bifida, in the newborn baby. It is also a good source of vitamin K, which helps promote bone formation; adequate vitamin K levels in the diet help to limit neuronal damage in the brain and so are useful in the treatment of patients suffering from Alzheimer's disease, dementia from other causes, multiple sclerosis and Parkinson's disease.

Ashitaba *(Angelica keiskei koidzmi)*

The Japanese name 'ashitaba' means 'tomorrow's leaf' or 'earth growth' in English and refers to the fact that, if this plant's leaves are picked in the morning, new leaves will be in place by the next morning. Ashitaba is a 'super food' which has been consumed as a vegetable and medicine for many hundreds of years by the inhabitants of seven islands of Izu (the Longevity Islands). It is an Asian green vegetable that is rich in the highly potent antioxidants known as chalcones.

Chalcones are often responsible for the yellow pigment in many types of flowers, such as daisies and sunflowers. They are a class of flavonoid compounds which protect cells from the free-radical damage that is associated with the ageing process and many disorders, including cancer, as well as degenerative diseases. They also suppress the excessive secretion of gastric juice in the stomach, which is often caused by stress and can contribute to stomach ulcer formation. They help strengthen the immune system, regulate blood pressure and cholesterol levels and exhibit antiviral and antibacterial activities.

Chalcones have also been found to stimulate the production of nerve growth factor (NGF), which is essential in the development and survival of certain neurons (nerve cells) in the peripheral and central nervous system and hence reduce symptoms of Alzheimer's disease.

Most plants are devoid of vitamin B12, which is normally only obtainable through meat, fish and eggs. However, ashitaba, like barley grass, is a good source, making it an ideal supplement for vegetarians who omit these foods from their diet. A shortage of B12 can cause serious cognitive and nervous system problems, in addition to increasing the risk of cardiovascular disease and pernicious anaemia.

Asparagus *(Asparagus officinalis)*
Asparagus is a member of the lily family and grows easily in the home garden right in the flower bed. It is a perennial and can yield a harvest for decades. It can be planted as seeds or roots at any time of the year. Regular consumption can help to reduce belly fat, prevent and remedy urinary tract infections and kidney stones and reduce pain and inflammation. In addition, it has anti-ageing properties and

will reduce the risk of heart disease as it protects blood cholesterol from peroxidation.

Specific components in asparagus can also prevent cellular damage that can lead to cancer and heart disease and can reduce the accumulation of iron in the joints, which is thought to be a primary cause of rheumatoid arthritis. There have been cases where asparagus has been able to eliminate cancerous tumours in the body completely. This may be due to its ability to reduce the accumulation of iron in the body because cancerous cells need iron to multiply. Asparagus's antioxidant properties and vitamin K content are additional anti-cancer agents so regular consumption (allowing for seasonality) is obviously beneficial to both protect against and treat cancer.

Because of its high vitamin B9 (folate) content, asparagus is useful for women who are pregnant or plan to become pregnant to prevent spina bifida (spinal cord birth defect) and also anencephaly (another neural tube defect). The rich content of vitamin B9 helps to regulate embryonic and foetal nerve cell formation and may also help to prevent premature births.

Aubergine *(Solanum melongena,* eggplant - nightshade family*)*

Aubergines can be grown in the ground or in pots and containers and just three plants will keep a family of four supplied with aubergines from mid-summer to late autumn. In addition to featuring a host of vitamins and minerals, aubergine also contains important phytonutrients, many of which have antioxidant activity, including caffeic and chlorogenic acid, and flavonoids, such as nasunin.

Chlorogenic acid has anti-mutagenic (anti-cancer), antimicrobial and antiviral properties and can lower LDL cholesterol. Nasunin has been shown to protect cell membranes from damage, especially the lipids (fats) in brain cell membranes. Cell membranes are almost entirely composed of lipids and are responsible for protecting the cell from free radicals, letting nutrients in and wastes out and receiving instructions from messenger molecules that tell the cell which activities it should perform. Thus aubergines are good for the brain cells.

The anthocyanins, in the purple skin of aubergines, can help to slow down age-related motor changes, such as those seen in Alzheimer's or Parkinson's disease, and prevent the oxidation of certain compounds and fight attacks on the body from harmful chemicals. They also increase vitamin C levels within cells, decrease the breakage of small blood vessels, protect against free-radical damage and help prevent destruction of collagen (the tissues under the skin) by helping the collagen fibres link together in a way that strengthens the connective tissue matrix.

They also reduce blood glucose levels and improve insulin sensitivity due to their ability to reduce the level of retinol-binding protein 4 (RBP4) in the blood. Elevated levels of this correlate with cardiovascular disease and diabetic retinopathy, so regular consumption of aubergines is useful in preventing diabetes and heart disease and can help with treating obesity.

Beans *(Fabaceae)*

Beans, like peas, are part of the family known as legumes - plants with seed pods that split into two halves. They are easily grown in pots or the ground but need support from canes or sticks and growing sweet peas amongst them can help to attract the insect pollinators needed to increase the yield. They can be started off indoors and planted out after the frosts have gone and are very easy to take care of but do need plenty of water and should be fed weekly (see page 95) once the first flowers set.

All types of legumes can reduce the risk of heart disease, lower LDL cholesterol, control blood sugar levels, lower the risks of colon cancer, prevent anaemia and maintain the proper levels of iron and calcium in the body. Because they are low in fat and cholesterol levels, but rich in protein, they are a useful alternative to balance the diet when meat and dairy products are reduced in the diet.

It was 7000 years ago, when the Hoabinhian people first cultivated the broad bean (*Vicia faba*), as was discovered by the seeds found in the Spirit Cave in Thailand. Broad beans remained a popular crop and the seeds are mentioned in Hittite and Ancient Egyptian sources dating from more than 3000 years ago, as well as in the Bible. They are one of the beans that do not grow very tall but do need some support and feeding (see page 93) once the first flowers have set.

Broad beans contain high amounts of levodopa, which is converted to the neurotransmitters epinephrine (adrenaline), dopamine and norepinephrine (noradrenaline) by the enzyme tyrosine hydroxylase in the brain. Levodopa, phenylalanine and tyrosine are precursors to the biological pigment melanin which determines eye, hair and skin colour. Regular consumption of broad beans may help those suffering from Parkinson's disease and also help to protect against skin cancer.

Fresh green beans (*Phaseolus vulgaris*), also known as runner beans, string beans, French beans, wax beans and pole beans, are very low in calories (31 kcal per 100 grams of raw beans) and contain no saturated fat. They are also a very rich source of dietary fibre and contain excellent levels of vitamin A, and the health-promoting flavonoid antioxidants beta-carotene, lutein and zeaxanthin. Zeaxanthin is selectively absorbed into the part of the retina called the macula lutea in the eyes, so green beans offer some protection in preventing age-related macular degeneration in the elderly. Green beans also help to control heart rate and blood pressure and reduce LDL cholesterol levels.

Green beans also provide vitamin B9, which, along with vitamin B12, is one of the essential components of DNA synthesis and cell division and, when consumed during preconception periods and pregnancy, helps prevent neural tube defects in the developing foetus.

Beetroot *(Beta vulgaris)*

Beetroot are very easy to grow for the novice gardener but must be grown in stone-free soil and do not do well if manure has been recently added to the soil. The leaves and roots are both edible and highly nutritious.

Beetroot are ideal for treating anaemia. With its high iron content, beetroot juice regenerates and reactivates the red blood cells, supplies the body with fresh oxygen and helps the normal function of vesicular breathing. Beetroot also helps prevent spina bifida in babies when consumed before and during pregnancy.

Regular consumption also reduces the risk of heart disease, helps control cholesterol levels, stops the spread of cancerous tumours, prevents diseases of liver, kidney and pancreas and treats ulcers in the stomach. It also strengthens the immune system, improves vision and is good for eye redness treatment.

Consuming beetroot can reduce pain after intense physical training and is a useful refuelling food for tired muscles. It also positively affects the colon and eliminates hard stools, strengthens the lungs, regulates blood pressure, improves bad breath, creates healthy skin, helps to treat acne and reduces menstrual pain. Beetroot possess the antioxidant beta-cyanin, which gives them their deep red colour and can assist the body with recovery from many ailments.

Bell peppers *(Capsicum annuum,* nightshade family*)*

Bell peppers are one of the easiest food crops to grow and all colours - green, red, orange or yellow - are rich sources of some of the best nutrients available. They are excellent sources of vitamins C and A (through the concentration of carotenoids, such as beta-carotene) which are two very powerful antioxidants that work together to effectively neutralise free radicals, which can travel through the body causing great damage to cells.

Free radicals can also cause the build-up of cholesterol in the arteries, which leads to atherosclerosis and heart disease, the nerve and blood vessel damage seen in diabetes, the cloudy lenses of cataracts, the joint pain and damage seen in osteoarthritis and rheumatoid arthritis and the wheezing and airway tightening of asthma.

Red peppers, like tomatoes, are one of the few foods that contain lycopene, a carotenoid whose consumption has been proven to reduce the risk of bladder, cervix, pancreas and prostate cancers. Tobacco smokers who regularly consume red bell peppers are less likely to develop lung cancer due to the beta-carotene, cryptoxanthin and lycopene content. Smokers are often deficient in vitamin A.

There are also compounds in bell peppers that protect against cataracts and macular degeneration, the main cause of blindness in the elderly.

Brassicas *(Brassicaceae, cruciferae,* cruciferous vegetables*)*

The word 'brassica' comes from 'bresic', a Celtic word for cabbage, and plants were originally named brassicas for the four equal-sized petals in their flowers that could be viewed as forming a cross-like or crucifix shape which is why they are also called cruciferous vegetables. Brassicas are all fairly simple to grow but do need plenty of feeding (see page 95) and to be kept well-watered and they can be attacked by various pests so need to be protected.

Glucoraphanin, which transforms into sulforaphane in the body, is found in brassicas and blocks a key destructive enzyme that damages cartilage. Regular consumption of brassicas can protect the joints and help to treat arthritis. Sulforaphane also helps with detoxification in the liver and may prevent, or even help to cure, breast cancer.

Brassicas can boost the immune system, prevent spina bifida in newborns (if consumed before and during pregnancy) and prevent heart disease and many forms of cancer. They also have a very high antioxidant content which cleanses the system and protects the lungs, and their high carotenoid and vitamin A content can protect the eyes. See the list of vegetables that are in brassica family on page 95.

NOTE: To benefit from the fat-soluble carotenoids in brassicas, they must be consumed with a fatty food such as avocado, coconut oil, fish oils and nut, seed and other cold-pressed plant oils.

Carrots *(Daucus carota)*

Carrots can be grown in a container that is more than two feet deep, such as a plastic refuse bin, as the carrot flies that attack them cannot fly higher than two feet above the ground. Cut some holes in the bottom of the large bin then add a layer of stones or broken pots for drainage. Then add sieved stone-free soil and top with a good potting compost before sowing your organic carrot seeds. Grow some spring onions around the edges to provide even more protection.

Carrots are an excellent source of antioxidant compounds and one of the richest sources of the pro-vitamin A, carotenoids. Carrots' antioxidant compounds help protect against cardiovascular disease and cancer and also promote good eyesight, especially night vision. They can also prevent blood clots and arterial blockages, reducing the risks of heart disease and strokes. They also prevent a variety of cancers and protect against the damage caused by nicotine. In addition, they are high in anti-ageing vitamin C and a good source of dietary fibre. Eating two carrots a day can lower cholesterol levels by 10%.

The raw juice of parsley, carrots and celery is very valuable as nourishment for the optic system, also for the kidneys and bladder and as an aid in allaying inflammation of the urethra and genital organs.

Celery *(Apium graveolens)*

Celery grows very easily but needs plenty of watering and a sunny spot. It is very low in calories so is useful for those trying to lose weight. It also relieves high blood pressure, is known for its calming effect and is used in the treatment of rheumatoid arthritis.

For many years, researchers and practitioners have been interested in the healing properties of celery seeds because they were documented as a natural pain reliever as far back as 30 AD in the Roman text *De Medicina*. Scientists have now identified the active ingredients in celery seeds, known as phthalides (pronounced 'thalides'). This compound has been shown to help prevent and treat arthritis, asthma, gall stones, gout, heart attack, kidney and bladder stones and strokes. It can act as a diuretic to reduce fluids, improve circulation, promote cleansing of toxins such as uric acid, reduce inflammation and relax the walls of arteries and veins. It also has antiviral properties.

Chilli peppers *(Capsicum anuum,* nightshade family*)*

Chilli pepper is a gift to humanity because it has more health benefits than any other food or herb on earth. There are over 3000 scientific studies listed in the National Library of Medicine to support the use of chilli pepper in preventing and reversing many common health ailments. It has been used as a food, a spice and a herbal medicine for over 9000 years and is probably one of the easiest food crops to grow in a pot.

The capsaicin in chilli peppers has been proven to protect DNA and cells from attack by toxic molecules from tobacco and other ingested products. It can also prevent cancer by inhibiting the transformation of cells which eventually form cancer.

Some of the conditions which chilli can be used to treat are allergies, arthritis, asthma, bacterial infections, blood circulation problems, cancer, colds and 'flu, constipation, depression, diabetes, diminished vitality, haemorrhoids, headaches, heart disease, high blood pressure, high cholesterol, indigestion, obesity, osteoarthritis and stroke.

It also nourishes the digestive system and assists in the body's utilisation of other herbs, when used in a herbal combination. Chilli pepper has benefits for the circulatory system and helps to balance blood pressure and resist abnormal bleeding.

To benefit from chilli peppers' powerful components, stir a quarter teaspoon of chilli pepper in water, herbal teas or juice and drink it one to three times a day or add a pinch of chilli pepper to all meals. Chilli pepper is hot, but not harmful, although it may be difficult to swallow at first.

When applied topically, it helps relieve minor discomfort and can stop bleeding (internally and externally). Chilli powder can also be rubbed on toothaches, swellings and inflammations. A remedy for arthritis is to rub a little chilli pepper over the inflamed joint and wrap a flannel around it to remain throughout the night. The pain is usually relieved by the morning. A little chilli pepper on a banana skin placed on the skin with a bandage will remarkably draw out any foreign object (splinters, etc) embedded in the flesh.

For a bleeding wound, liberally flush the wound with a chilli pepper tincture or pack with chilli powder and apply pressure to the wound. Depending on the severity of the bleeding, also take one to 10 droppers full of the tincture in a few ounces of water in the mouth. **NOTE**: It is said that chilli pepper can work as quickly as a soluble aspirin in an emergency when someone is suffering a heart attack. However, there is no scientific proof that this is possible and it can be dangerous to administer chilli pepper to someone who is suffering from a heart attack. Experts say its use could lead to uncontrolled bleeding if the person is taking blood-thinning medications and the pain of ingesting a dose of hot pepper could cause adrenaline to be released, increasing heart rate while reducing blood flow to heart and brain, which will cause increased death of tissues. Reperfusion injuries (damage to tissues from the sudden return of blood and oxygen), could also occur. Some websites actually encourage the administration of liquid cayenne extracts to heart attack victims who have lost consciousness, which is very dangerous advice.

Courgettes *(Cucurbita pepo,* zucchini)
Courgettes are one of the easiest food crops to grow and one plant will

provide enough for a family of four from early summer to autumn. Some varieties can be harvested within six weeks of planting. They will need support or can be grown like other vines, such as pumpkins, in a raised bed. They are very easy to take care of but do need plenty of water and should be fed (see page 95) weekly once the first flowers set. The flowers make colourful and edible decorations for salads.

The courgette is one of the lowest calorie vegetables with only 17 calories per 100 grams and contains no saturated fats or cholesterol so is ideal for those trying to lose weight. Its peel is a good source of dietary fibre that helps reduce constipation and can prevent colon cancers. Because dietary fibre promotes healthy and regular bowel movements it also helps to prevent carcinogenic toxins from settling in the colon. Dietary fibre also binds well with bile acid, thus crowding its ability to immediately digest fat. The liver is then forced to produce more bile acid, which makes it draw upon even more cholesterol, consequently lowering the overall cholesterol level in the body. Also the high levels of vitamin A and C prevent cholesterol from oxidising in the body's blood vessels, thus hampering the onset of atherosclerosis (blood vessel damage).

The nutrients in courgettes can fight many different types of cancer and deter the development of many disorders, including asthma, heart attack, irritable bowel syndrome, osteoarthritis, rheumatoid arthritis, stomach disorders and stroke and can protect the eyes. They also lower blood pressure, contribute to normal physiological functions, participate in the production of sex hormones, protect mitochondria against oxidative stress and promote healthy skin and proper wound-healing. There are also components in courgettes that help in reducing the symptoms of benign prostatic hypertrophy, a condition in which the prostate gland enlarges and leads to complications with urination and sexual function in men.

Cucumber *(Cucumis sativus)*

Some types of cucumber can easily be grown outside in containers or in the ground and will produce about 10 to 15 fruits per plant. Other species need to be grown in a greenhouse or conservatory and these indoor varieties will need to have the male flowers removed or they will fertilise the fruits which will then taste bitter. They will need feeding and plenty of water once the flowers have set.

The cucumber's hard skin is rich in fibre and contains a variety of beneficial minerals, including potassium, magnesium and silica; the latter is an essential component of healthy connective tissue, which includes intracellular cement, muscles, tendons, ligaments, cartilage and bone. Cucumber juice is often recommended as a source of silica to improve the complexion and health of the skin, including swelling under the eyes and sunburn, plus cucumber's high-water content makes it naturally hydrating. The flesh of cucumbers is primarily composed of water but also contains vitamin C and caffeic acid, both of which help soothe skin irritations and reduce swelling. Cucumbers also possess cancer-preventing and anti-tumour properties and reduce body weight, lipid metabolism and obesity-related hormone levels.

Fenugreek *(Trigonella foenum)*

Fenugreek is very easy to grow from seed. The seeds need to be soaked overnight and then sprinkled onto soil or in a pot or container. They will begin to sprout within a couple of days. Fenugreek greens, known as 'methi', either fresh or dried, are highly nutritious and one of the prominent leafy-greens featured in Indian and Pakistani cooking, with spinach, potato (aaloomethi) and carrots etc.

Fenugreek seeds have many medicinal uses, including nourishing the skin, respiratory system and pancreas. They also help the body to expel mucus and toxins and dissolve fat and are also high in nutrients. They are a very good source of soluble dietary fibre; soaking the seeds in water makes their outer coat soft and mucilaginous, similar to chia seeds. Altogether 100 grams of seeds provide 24.6 grams, or over 65%, of the daily requirement for dietary fibre. Fenugreek seeds added to cereals and wheat flour (bread) or made into porridge and given to nursing mothers, may increase breast milk production.

Fenugreek can also be used to control diabetes, improve glucose tolerance and lower blood sugar levels due to its hypoglycaemic activity as it stimulates the secretion of glucose-dependent insulin. Being high in fibre, it also slows down the absorption of carbohydrates and sugars. Soak two tablespoons of fenugreek seeds in water overnight. Drink the water along with the seeds in the morning on an empty stomach. Follow this remedy for a few months to bring down glucose levels. Another option is to eat two tablespoons of powdered fenugreek seeds daily, sprinkled onto meals.

Garlic *(Allium sativa)*

Garlic grows well in the ground in soil with good drainage as well as in containers indoors or outside. It is a slow-growing root vegetable but its exceptional medicinal properties are well worth the wait. Garlic provides nourishment for the circulatory, immune and urinary systems. It helps in supporting stomach tissues, maintaining normal blood pressure and the body's natural ability to resist disease. It also helps to reduce cholesterol and fat deposits. It is a natural antibiotic, antimicrobial and an antioxidant. It is also a blood purifier, detoxifies the liver and protects against tumours and stomach cancer.

Consuming three garlic cloves per day can provide health maintenance and more if there is an existing health issue. Always leave garlic to stand for 10 minutes after chopping or crushing to allow the powerful and protective allicin compound to be produced. Health issues garlic can help to treat include:

- Arthritis
- Asthma
- Bacterial infections
- Bronchitis
- Cancer
- Candida
- Colds
- Colitis
- Coughs
- Digestive problems
- Fever
- Flatulence
- Fungal infections
- High blood pressure
- Influenza
- Intestinal infections
- Liver disorders
- Lung disorders
- Parasitic diarrhoea
- Poor circulation
- Sore throat
- Toothache

- *Toxoplasmosis gondii* infection
- Viruses
- Warts
- Whooping cough
- Worms and parasites
- Yeast infections

Leeks *(Allium porrum)*

Leeks have a reputation of being difficult to grow when in fact they are easily grown from seed and will provide a harvest from November right through to the following March, and most species will survive the coldest winters.

A flavonoid called kaempferol is present in significant amounts in leeks and this provides protection to the linings of the blood vessels, particularly against free radicals. Kaempferol also induces the increased production of nitric oxide, a substance that acts as a natural dilator and relaxant of the blood vessels and therefore decreases the risk of hypertension (high blood pressure). Leeks are also a good source of vitamin C, vitamin B6, vitamin K, manganese and iron.

Okra *(Abelmoschus esculentus,* lady fingers, gumbo*)*

Okra is a perennial flowering plant that belongs to the mallow family and the green edible pods are highly nutritious. It needs plenty of sun but also shelter from wind, and grows best under glass. Okra pods are very low-calorie vegetables, providing just 30 calories per 100 grams, and contain no saturated fats or cholesterol. The rich fibre and mucilaginous content in okra pods help achieve smooth peristalsis of digested food particles and relieve constipation.

This is a supreme vegetable for those feeling weak, exhausted and suffering from depression. It feeds the beneficial bacteria in the guts, binds to excess cholesterol and toxins and eliminates them through the stools. It also stabilises cholesterol and blood sugar levels to provide good protection against heart disease and diabetes. It is good for the vision and lowers the risk of cataracts. It also maintains healthy mucous membranes and skin, treats acne, helps to develop immunity against infectious agents, reduces episodes of asthma, colds and coughs, strengthens the bones, may remedy lung inflammation, sore throat and irritable bowel syndrome and helps to protect against colon, liver, kidney, lung and oral cavity cancers.

Onion *(Allium cepa)*
Onions are easy to take care of but they do need free-draining soil. Harvest onions a week or two after the leaves begin to turn yellow. Choose a dry day to loosen them from the ground, then leave them on the soil surface for a couple of days until they have fully dried in the sun. Regular consumption of onions can help to prevent cancer, circulatory disorders, diabetes and heart disease and they are particularly useful in reducing the development of bladder cancer in smokers. Onions contain vitamin C, vitamin K, vitamin B9 (folic acid), chromium, quercetin and allicin.

Allicin is produced by plants in the onion family when they are damaged to help protect them and also has powerful antimicrobial and tumour-fighting properties in the human body when consumed.

It can help to reduce atherosclerosis and fat deposition, normalise the lipoprotein balance, decrease blood pressure, has anti-inflammatory activities and functions as an antioxidant.

NOTE: The onion family includes chives, garlic, leeks, shallots and spring onions. Always leave plants from the onion family for 10 minutes after chopping them to allow the production of allicin to take place. Once they are being cooked this ceases.

Parsnips *(Pastinaca sativa)*

Parsnips are as easy to grow as carrots and potatoes but take a little longer to be ready for harvesting. However, they contain far more heart-friendly potassium and vitamin B9 than carrots and more soluble and insoluble fibre than potatoes. Vitamin B9 is required for the creation of healthy cells and having insufficient levels has been linked to birth defects and cancer. Adequate fibre in the diet helps reduce blood cholesterol levels and obesity and can alleviate constipation.

Parsnips are also a rich source of manganese, which is required by the nerves and brain, aids the coordination of nerve impulses and muscular actions, and helps to eliminate fatigue and reduce nervous irritability. Parsnip leaves and stalks are also edible and beneficial for remedyinging asthma and cancer.

NOTE: In Europe, parsnips were used to sweeten jams and cakes before sugar was widely available and this is a far healthier alternative.

Peas *(Pisum sativum)*

Peas like fertile, rich soil so compost should be added before planting the pea seeds. Sweet peas should be grown with them to attract pollinating insects. They are very easy to take care of but do need plenty of water and should be fed weekly once the first flowers set.

Peas are a rich source of the powerful antioxidant alpha-lipoic acid that has the ability to rehabilitate other antioxidants, such as glutathione and vitamins C and E, which tend to wear themselves out and dissipate. Alpha-lipoic acid also helps the body use glucose; hence, it is useful in lowering blood sugar levels and in the management of diabetes and may help prevent the cellular damage accompanying the complications of diabetes. It also has a protective effect on the brain and nerve tissues.

Potatoes *(Solanum tuberosum,* nightshade family*)*

Potatoes are among the 12 foods on which pesticide residues have been most frequently found and therefore it is useful to grow your own organically. The potato belongs to the nightshade family whose other members include tomatoes, aubergines and peppers. They are an easy and excellent first crop to grow as they break up the soil and improve its mineral content.

Potatoes are useful for easing colic, constipation, gastritis, indigestion and stomach ulcers. Externally, they are useful for chilblains, inflamed skin, minor burns, skin infections, sunburn and even headaches.

It is important to grow potatoes in a wide enough space so that soil can be pushed up over them as they grow.

White potatoes that have turned green and the potato leaves contain a compound called solanine which is poisonous. Solanine is a steroid glycoside of the saponin group found in plants from the nightshade family which, in large doses, can cause gastrointestinal disorders such as diarrhoea and vomiting, hallucinations, paralysis and death. One of the triggers for solanine to develop in a white potato is exposure to light, especially fluorescent light. Therefore, it is essential to store harvested potatoes in a dark place, preferably between 10°C and 18°C (50°F and 65°F). If potatoes must be stored in a lighted place, they can be kept in a brown paper bag loosely closed to allow for air circulation.

Pumpkin *(Curcubita pepo)*

Pumpkins do require a lot of food (see page 95) and a long growing season, generally from 85 to 125 frost-free days as this is how long they take to mature. They are vines that will take up quite a bit of space but the health benefits of both pumpkins and their seeds are immense.

Pumpkin, especially the seeds, protects skin and mucous membranes from the ageing effects of free radicals (page 21) and contributes to the health of the retina and lens of the eye. It also maintains optimum thyroid function and blood sugar levels, lowers LDL ('bad') cholesterol levels, increases HDL ('good') cholesterol levels, is good for bone and nerve health and protects against osteoporosis, strokes and coronary heart disease. Regular consumption is also therapeutic to those afflicted with arthritis, bladder and urinary problems and can protect against cancers, such as prostate, breast, lung, ovarian, and stomach and improves the immune response.

Pumpkin seeds, also known as 'pepitas', have important health benefits for men, as they have properties that can inhibit prostate cell multiplication. This may be due to the high zinc, omega-3 fatty acid, phytosterol and carotenoid content. Tryptophan is also abundant in pumpkin seeds, which can relieve anxiety and depression, and the powerful anti-inflammatory properties of these seeds has been shown to do better than anti-inflammatory drugs without the negative side effects. Consume a handful of seeds daily to acquire all the above health benefits.

Radish *(Raphanus sativus)*

Radishes are members of the brassica family and can be white, red, purple or black. They are very easy to grow as they tolerate most soil types and are quick to crop (usually within three weeks). Because of this they should be planted in small batches each week for a constant harvest.

Radishes contain a volatile ether which is particularly useful as a solvent for mucus or phlegm. They have also enzymes valuable in aiding the secretion of digestive juices and, because of their diuretic action, they are valuable in cleansing the kidneys and the bladder. The juice of radishes blended with carrot juice is a wonderful aid in cleansing and healing the mucous membrane of the digestive system as well as of the respiratory organs.

Radish is very good for the liver and is an excellent detoxifier to purify the blood. It is useful for remedying jaundice as it helps remove bilirubin and also checks its production. It also checks destruction of red blood cells during jaundice by increasing supply of fresh oxygen in the blood. The black radish and radish leaves generally are best for this purpose.

Regular consumption of radishes can help to relieve and remedy asthma, bronchitis, constipation, fever, gall bladder problems, kidney and liver disorders, haemorrhoids (piles), respiratory disorders, urinary tract infections, skin disorders and many forms of cancer. They are also useful for weight loss and can be used externally for insect bites.

Spinach *(Spinacia oleracea)*

Spinach is a member of the brassica family and a very easy, fast-growing and nutritious food crop. It can even be grown indoors on a windowsill during the winter. Regular consumption of spinach can protect against arthritis, asthma, colon cancer, heart disease, osteoporosis, prostate cancer and rheumatoid arthritis. It is an exceptionally rich source of vitamin K2 that can activate osteocalcin, the major non-collagen protein in bone. The high amounts of magnesium and vitamin B2 (riboflavin) can help to prevent migraines.

There are also compounds in spinach that can improve the learning capacity and motor skills and significantly lessen brain damage from strokes and other neurological disorders. Cooked spinach is an excellent source of iron which is important for menstruating women who are at risk of iron deficiency. During pregnancy and breast feeding the need for iron increases and growing children and adolescents also have increased needs for iron.

Spring onions *(Alliaceae)*

Spring onions are very simple to grow in clumps anywhere, including pots and containers, and are useful to plant amongst other vegetables as they can deter aphids and other pests. The green stalks of spring onions should always be consumed too as, like all leafy greens, they contain nutrients such as chlorophyll which is the green pigment present in plants and is a molecule that absorbs sunlight and uses its energy to synthesise carbohydrates from CO_2 and water in a process known as photosynthesis. Because the chlorophyll molecule is almost identical to the haemoglobin molecule in red blood cells it is often referred to as 'nature's blood'.

One of chlorophyll's many attributes includes its ability to stimulate the production of red blood cells, which carry oxygen to the body's tissues. It is also an excellent agent for cleansing the blood, bowels and liver and promotes the growth of beneficial intestinal bacteria. It can also bind with heavy metals and remove them from the body and strengthens immunity. In addition It also has antioxidant and anti-inflammatory properties, alkalises the blood, helps fight off diseases and protects against cancer.

Swede *(Brassica napus,* rutabaga*)*

Swedes are one of the easiest vegetables to grow for a novice gardener and, although they take some time to mature ready for harvest, they are worth the wait. They do need very free-draining soil, though or they will rot.

Regular consumption of swede can increase milk production capacity in lactating mothers. It also can increase and enhance digestion and stamina. Swede also helps in reducing wheezing in asthma patients and the risk of cataract formation, supports the structure of capillaries, helps in decreasing stroke mortality, can lower high blood pressure and provides relief from constipation.

In addition, swede boosts the immune system, prevents cancer and heart disease and, when consumed by women, before and during pregnancy, it can prevent spina bifida in the newborn baby. Swede is also good to include in the diet when suffering from colds and coughs.

Sweet corn *(Zea mays,* Indian corn, jugnog, maize, sea mays, yu-shu-shu*)*

Sweetcorn is a good organic food crop to grow because so many commercially produced varieties have now been tampered with by genetic modification and whether this is positive or negative for health and the environment is still being debated. It is very easy to grow, but does require regular feeding, watering and space, needing at least 12 plants planted in a block to produce cobs successfully.

Sweetcorn is high in fibre, which can help with digestion or colon disorders. It is also a very good source of vitamin B9 which helps to lower levels of the amino acid homocysteine. Homocysteine can directly damage blood vessels, so elevated blood levels of this dangerous molecule are a risk factor for heart attack, stroke and peripheral vascular disease. Vitamin B9 (folate) also lowers the risk of spina bifida in babies if consumed by women before and during pregnancy. Sweetcorn can help to balance blood sugar levels while providing steady, slow-burning energy so is a useful food for those with diabetes type 2.

Corn silk refers to the stigmas from the female flowers of sweet corn and resembles soft silk threads 10-20 cm long that are either light green or yellow-brown in colour. A tea made from corn silk is useful as a diuretic and has been said to help disorders of the bladder, gallbladder, kidneys, liver and small intestines, such as bed-wetting, bladder and kidney stones, cystitis, jaundice, painful urination caused by an enlarged prostate gland, pancreatic damage and urinary tract infection. It is also useful for the treatment of diabetes type 2, dropsy, gonorrhoea, gout, heart disease, hypertension (high blood pressure), oedema (water retention) and rheumatism.

Sweet potato *(Ipomoea batatas)*

Sweet potatoes only thrive in warmer temperate climates and loose sandy soil that is well drained and only produce seed in tropical climates. In northern climates, new plants are obtained by planting roots, or cuttings of the vines, in beds. The sprouts that form are then replanted in a field, one sprout to a 'hill' of soil. Once they are established, they require very little watering and, unless attacked by the numerous diseases and insect pests to which they are subject, develop many potatoes in each hill. Sweet potatoes produce more pounds of food per acre than any other cultivated plant, including corn and the white potato.

Because white potatoes are members of the nightshade family, which some people have intolerances to, sweet potatoes are a good substitute. Although some people call sweet potatoes yams, the true yam originated in China and is a different plant, related to the lily.

Sweet potato contains no saturated fats or cholesterol and provides 90 calories per 100 grams whereas white potato contains 70 calories per 100. They also contain more fibre, iron, vitamins C, B9 and K2 and potassium but less sodium than the white potato.

The anti-oxidants beta-carotene, manganese, selenium and vitamins A, C and E in sweet potatoes can improve the condition of the skin and hair and help to treat arthritis, asthma and gout. Most smokers have a lack of vitamin A and have problems with emphysema (air sac damage). Sweet potatoes rejuvenate the respiratory system and prevent emphysema because of the high amounts of carotenoids that they contain. A 100-gram tuber provides 19218 μg (micrograms) of vitamin A and 8509 μg of beta-carotene, the precursor to vitamin A. Vitamin A is required by the body to maintain the integrity of healthy skin and the mucous membranes that line the organs of the body.

The anthocyanins in the purple-skinned sweet potato varieties can remove wrinkles and dark circles around the eyes and help to reduce puffy and swollen eyes. After boiling the potatoes with their skins on, keep the water and use it to clean the face for blemish-free, healthy skin.

Because they contain iron and help with the production of red and white blood cells, sweet potatoes can prevent and treat anaemia. The magnesium and iron also help to treat menstrual symptoms, both before and during menstruation. Sweet potatoes can control and maintain normal blood pressure and balance the levels of minerals in the body due to their high potassium content. The high amount of vitamin B6 helps the function of the heart and prevents heart attacks, strokes and digestive issues.

The vitamin D can help to support the immune system and is very important for maintaining the health of the thyroid gland, bones, teeth, skin and heart. Sweet potatoes also contain high amounts of magnesium that helps the whole body system and functions as an anti-stress agent. Other components can help to normalise the heart beat and the nerve signals that are sent to the brain. The minerals germanium and selenium also help to build muscles and prevent muscle cramps and minimise swelling.

Sweet potatoes contain natural sugar which controls and stabilises sugar levels in the blood. Not only do they have a low glycaemic index (the measure of how quickly a food raises blood sugar), but they have been shown in a clinical trial to help reduce blood sugar levels and improve insulin sensitivity in adults with type II diabetes. This may be due to their chromium content. The vitamin A in sweet potatoes can help to prevent retinal disorders, which are common in people with diabetes. One study has shown that sweet potatoes reduce appetite and food intake, which can help those trying to lose weight.

In 1931, a unique protein, known as sporamin, was discovered in sweet potatoes and it was found that 80% of the protein in sweet potatoes is this type of protease inhibitor that has powerful anticancer effects. It was first tried on tongue cancer with very favourable results and further studies showed it has the ability to slow the growth of colon cancer cells by 65%. It also inhibited lung and oral cancers by 50%. Other lab research has shown that sweet potato protein also potently inhibits leukaemia, lymphoma and liver cancer cells, and in studies on humans, eating this vegetable, either alone or with other foods, has been associated with reducing the risk of kidney cancer by 56%, gallbladder cancer by 67% and breast cancer by 30%, when consumed three times a week. The purple skins of sweet potatoes are rich in flavonoids which also help to protect against all these cancers.

Sweet potatoes contain high amounts of dietary fibre and thus prevent constipation and colon cancer and they are extremely beneficial to consume during pregnancy because they have high levels of vitamin B9 which is necessary for foetal tissue health maintenance and the prevention of neural tube defects, such as spina bifida.

Swiss chard *(Beta vulgaris)*

Swiss chard are the leaves and stems of a species of the beetroot plant and are very easy to grow but do need plenty of sunshine and watering. They can be grown in a container and provide their colourful stems and green leaves all summer long if planted in successions.

Swiss chard contains at least 13 different polyphenol antioxidants, including kaempferol, the cardio-protective flavonoid that is also found in broccoli, kale, strawberries and other food crops. Another of the flavonoids they contain is syringic acid which has powerful blood-sugar regulating properties. They also contain both red/purple betacyanin and yellow betaxanthin pigments which have been shown to provide antioxidant, anti-inflammatory and detoxification support for the body.

NOTE: Due to its oxalate content, individuals with already existing and untreated kidney or gallbladder problems may want to avoid eating Swiss chard.

Tomatoes *(Lycopersicon esculentum, Solanum lycopersicum, nightshade family)*

Tomatoes are one of the easiest crops to grow and thrive in the ground or containers but do need feeding weekly once the flowers have set. They are also very thirsty plants and an automatic watering system works best as they can quickly dry out and wilt, although, as long as you are vigilant and make sure to water them often and sometimes twice a day in hot weather, they will provide a huge crop that can last all through the winter. They must be harvested before the frosts arrive in autumn and, if they are still green simply hang the vine of tomatoes up near a sunny window and they will turn red.

Tomatoes are rich in many beneficial nutrients such beta-carotene, copper, lycopene, manganese, molybdenum, phosphorus, potassium and vitamins B3, B6, B7, B9, C, E and K. Regular consumption can lower the risk of breast, colon, mouth, oesophagus, pancreatic, prostate and stomach cancers and of developing asthma, atherosclerosis, diabetic complications and heart disease. They can also stimulate mental and physical activity in the elderly. Cooked tomatoes contain more antioxidants but the heating lowers the level of vitamin C.

Turnips and turnip greens *(Brassica rapa,* neep*)*

Turnips are very fast and easy to grow in stone-free, fertile soil with plenty of drainage, and can be ready to harvest after six weeks or so. For this reason, it is good to sow a few seeds each month, after the frosts have gone, to provide a continuous supply all summer.

Turnip greens are supercharged with many different nutrients and regular consumption can help prevent and heal a wide range of health conditions and bacterial infections. They are an excellent source of vitamin A (through their concentration of carotenoids such as beta-carotene), vitamin E and dietary fibre and are particularly useful for alleviating rheumatoid arthritis and atherosclerosis.

Regular consumption of turnip roots can help to prevent blood clots and arterial blockages hence reducing the risk of heart disease, and prevent a variety of cancers, especially colorectal. They also protect against the damage caused by smoking tobacco.

Herbs

Most herbs are easy to grow both in the ground and in pots and other containers, indoors or outside, and all of them possess volatile essential oils with powerful medicinal properties. Use herbs liberally in meals or make teas by steeping the leaves in hot water for 10 minutes, or boiling chopped up roots for 15 minutes before straining and drinking immediately. Three cups a day will generally provide all the medicinal benefits of herbs.

Adding the freshly squeezed juice of half a lemon and a pinch of black pepper will intensify their effects and a teaspoon of honey can be added if the taste is too bitter. Herbs and spices can be mixed together when more than one is required for any health issues. The beneficial components in herbs are more concentrated in the oil and seeds of plants. Seeds can be ground to release these components and added to meals or teas also.

NOTE: Essential oils of herbs are not suitable for pregnant or breastfeeding women or people with high blood pressure.

Basil *(Ocimum basilicum)*

Basil is one of the easiest herbs to grow, both indoors and outside, and complements many dishes, especially those that contain cheese or tomatoes. Components in basil have a balancing effect on the nervous system and hormones. A basil tea is good for lowering blood sugar levels and blood pressure and can treat difficult urination, fever, 'flu, hay fever, headache, kidney and bladder disorders, memory problems, migraines, nasal congestion and nervous conditions. It can also improve nutrient absorption and clear and relieve abdominal distension, congestion and respiratory disorders as it is analgesic and anti-inflammatory. Basil is antibiotic, antiseptic and an appetiser that benefits the stomach during digestion and can provide immediate relief from constipation, flatulence, indigestion, nausea, stomach cramps and vomiting.

The essential oil of basil contains eugenol, which works similarly to aspirin and ibuprofen in decreasing the swelling in joints and tissues to provide relief from arthritis, cramps, fibromyalgia, joint pain and rheumatism. Its powerful anti-inflammatory properties can also provide relief for inflamed bowel conditions, such as colitis, IBS, Crohn's disease and coeliac disease. Because of its antibacterial and antiviral properties, it is also effective against bacterial infections, intestinal parasites and the viruses that cause colds, 'flu, herpes, mononucleosis and shingles.

Basil is a rich source of magnesium, which relaxes muscles and blood vessels and supports cardiovascular health by lowering the risk of irregular heart rhythms and spasms. It can also help to strengthen nerve tissue, and is a heart tonic, oxygenates the body, cleanses the brain, relieves depression and the effects of poisons, prevents the accumulation of fat in the body (especially for women after menopause) and fights skin diseases, the first stages of many cancers and builds the immune system.

Make a tea with one large handful of leaves to 500 millilitres of water and simmer for 10 minutes. Then strain and add two crushed black peppercorns to each cupful. Three cups a day will be effective for all of the above health issues. Keep in the refrigerator for one day only. It can be reheated or drunk cold with lemon juice and ice.

Basil's fungicidal properties also help in healing wounds, rashes, warts and insect bites. Crush fresh leaves in a small amount of pure coconut oil, apply to the skin and wrap with a fresh bandage daily. Externally diluted essential oil can be useful for acne, hives, insect bites and skin infections. Basil can also work as a natural antihistamine to treat hives.

Borage *(Borago oficinalis)*

Borage is attractive to bees and butterflies and prefers full sun. It is excellent to grow alongside tomatoes and helps to improve a strawberry crop and, once established, the plants will return year after year. They do need to be grown in a container though as they spread very quickly. The leaves taste like cucumber and can be used as vegetable or in salads and the edible blue flowers can be added to summer drinks and salads; both are rich in many beneficial nutrients.

Borage seed oil contains gamma linolenic acid (GLA). GLA is a fatty acid the body converts to substances called prostaglandins, some of which have anti-inflammatory properties that are believed to act as blood thinners and blood vessel dilators. Borage oil also contains tannin antioxidants that protect the brain and neurons from oxidative stress. The combination of GLA and tannin antioxidants improves blood supply into the brain thereby providing more oxygen and nutrition into this vital structure. This oil can also reduce symptoms of rheumatoid arthritis and is useful for people with eczema.

Burdock *(Arctium lappa)*

Burdock is easily grown from seed and prefers a sandy garden soil in partial shade or full sun. It may be sown directly from early spring on into summer, with plenty of time left to get a good harvest of roots.

Burdock is the hardiest of root vegetables and winters in the garden easily for spring harvesting.

The root of the burdock plant is an excellent blood purifier and detoxifier. Very few, if any, herbs possess more curative powers than this one. It has an ancient history as a reliable herbal aid for blood disorders, ulcers, tumours and many skin diseases, such as acne, abscesses, dermatitis, eczema, furunculosis (boils), lupus, pityriasis and psoriasis. It also nutritionally supports joints and other skeletal tissues and the urinary and respiratory systems.

Burdock root also promotes glandular and hormone balance and removes accumulations and deposits around the joints. In addition, it is helpful against cancer, dyspeptic complaints, leprosy, liver and gall bladder problems, neurologic disorders, scrofula, syphilis and throat and chest ailments and expels toxic products from the blood through the urine. It is also an appetite stimulant and can control blood sugar and cholesterol levels, blood pressure, heart rate and weight and can help to prevent muscle wasting.

Chamomile *(Chamomilla recutita,* Roman chamomile, ground apple, whig plant*)*

Chamomile is a very easy herb to grow and does not require feeding in good soils. Some people use one particular species instead of a lawn for a green covering. Chamomile tea is made from the dried flower heads of the chamomile plant.

Chamomile is rich in aldehydes and sequiterpene that soothe the nerves and stomach. It also has components that support the respiratory tract and help alleviate discomfort associated with menstrual problems. It is also useful for treating gastrointestinal disorders, hay fever, inflammation, insomnia, muscle spasms and rheumatic pain. It can also inhibit the growth of *Helicobacter pylori* in the intestines

Three cups of chamomile tea a day will provide these benefits. To make tea, use about a teaspoon of dried chamomile flowers per cup. In the summer, ice cubes can be made to make a fresh iced tea. Freshly harvested chamomile can be used for tea as well, but will require twice as many flowers. Drying concentrates both the oils and flavour. Externally, chamomile tea can be used as a wash on the skin for inflammation and skin diseases.

Chicory *(Chihorium intybus, Cichorium endivia,* escarole, common chicory, blue sailors, succory, coffee weed, cornflower, endive, radicchio, Belgian endive, French endive, red endive, sugarloaf, witloof*)*

Chicory is an erect perennial herbaceous plant of the daisy family and related to the dandelion; it is good to grow it in containers due to its spreading fast, as they do. Chicory use in herbal medicine has a long history and some of its health benefits have recently been confirmed by science. The first recorded usage of it was in Ancient Egypt where it was known to support the liver and gall bladder. Chicory is prized for the leaves, roots and buds (chicons) which are all edible. The leaves and buds are used in salads and other dishes, while chicory roots are used as tea or a caffeine-free coffee substitute and additive.

It is very low in calories but highly nutritious and is one of the richest sources of vitamin A amongst all green leafy vegetables; vitamin A can nourish the eyes and improve and support the vision. Chicory leaves are also recommended to be included in weight-loss diets, especially for those who have a high risk of developing diabetes mellitus. The inulin content controls the level of sugar in the blood, decreases the level of LDL ('bad') cholesterol and reduces a rapid heartbeat.

Chicory roots contain inulin, which feeds the beneficial bacteria of the large intestine and these produce many beneficial substances, including short-chain fatty acids and certain B vitamins. They also promote further absorption of some minerals that have escaped the small intestine, including calcium and magnesium.

Chicory is rich in beta-carotene that can fight and prevent cancer, especially colon cancer, and also contains intybin and chicorin, which stimulate the appetite and digestion of food. It can also eliminate intestinal worms and parasites and clean the colon. In addition, it promotes the production of urine, cleans the blood, circulatory system and the liver by eliminating toxins from them, and improves bowel movement. It has a mild laxative effect that is beneficial for digestive problems such as dyspepsia, indigestion and constipation.

Dried chicory roots and leaf juice are used to treat jaundice and as protection against liver damage. The leaf juice mixed with water can clean up an enlarged liver and treat gallstones and liver stones by increasing the secretion of bile from the liver and gall bladder, promoting urination and excretion of harmful substances. Chicory roots also contain lactucin and lactucoprin, which taste bitter but can act as a natural sedative for the nervous system; a decoction of the root is beneficial for those with central nervous system disorders.

Chives *(Allium schoenoprasum)*
Chives grow well in pots indoors or outside and are useful for aphid control when placed near susceptible plants. Chives belong to the onion family and are fairly high in protein and carbohydrates and rich in calcium, potassium, phosphorus and sulphur. They are stimulating to the digestive system, valuable as a blood cleanser and exercise a strong diuretic action. The sulphur in chives can help to eliminate mercury when consumed with fish that may be contaminated by this toxin which has been accidently leaked into our oceans.
NOTE: Drinking beer should be avoided if consuming chives as it may cause undue discomfort.

Comfrey *(Symphytum officinale)*
Growing a patch of comfrey has many beneficial uses both for health and as a feed for other plants because it is adept at collecting potassium from the soil and distributing this around its leaves. Comfrey has components that can nourish the pituitary gland (the master gland of the body), as well as the bones and skin. It also strengthens the respiratory system and is considered to be one of nature's great healers.

Comfrey roots and leaves have a high concentration of mucilage that can be used to treat bronchitis, chronic coughs, diarrhoea, dysentery, glandular disorders, gout, irritable bowel syndrome, pulmonary haemorrhages, respiratory disorders and stomach ulcers. A tea made from comfrey can be used as a gargle to treat sore gums and throat hoarseness and, externally, it can be used as a compress to treat bronchitis, burns, gangrene, fibrosis, fractures, inflammation, mastitis, otitis, pleurisy, skin sores, sprains and varicose veins.

Coriander *(Coriandrum sativum,* cilantro)

Coriander can easily be grown in containers and the ground and seeds should be sown at three weekly intervals as it goes to seed very readily. For that reason, harvest the leaves often and then, when the plant flowers, leave the seeds to ripen and harvest those as well. The leaves are one of the main ingredients in salsa, along with tomatoes, onions and green chillies.

Both the leaves and seeds have effective medicinal properties and in parts of Europe, coriander has traditionally been referred to as an 'anti-diabetic' plant. In parts of India, it has traditionally been used for its anti-inflammatory properties as well as for digestive and gastric complaints, such as indigestion and nausea. It is also useful for bladder disorders, chest pains, chickenpox, coughs, dysentery, fever, halitosis, leprosy rash, oral and pharyngeal disorders, typhoid fever and complications after child birth.

Coriander leaves and seeds contain an antibacterial compound, dodecanal, that can be a safe, natural means of fighting *Salmonella* and also has a cholesterol-lowering effect. They also contain eight other antibiotic compounds that can prevent food-borne illness.

Coriander has been proven to be able to eliminate mercury from the body. Heavy metal contamination can lead to the development of conditions such as Alzheimer's, multiple sclerosis and Parkinson's disease. Adding some leaves to a dish which includes fish, which may have been contaminated by mercury, can help to prevent it from being absorbed by the body.

The seeds are useful to relieve fevers (a small amount of black pepper may be added to stimulate its action). Use two teaspoons of crushed seeds in a cup of boiled water and steep for 20 minutes. Coriander seeds used to be added to laxative formulas to help prevent cramping and, before the invention of toothpaste, they were chewed as a breath sweetener.

Dandelion *(Taraxacum officinale)*

The dandelion is probably one of the easiest plants to grow prolifically and for this reason must be grown in a container if you do not want it to spread everywhere. Although considered a weed and discarded from most gardens, the dandelion contains many vital nutrients that can help to protect the liver and kidneys. Dandelion root tea has been used traditionally to purify the blood and to benefit the circulatory and glandular systems and its compounds have natural diuretic properties. It stimulates the removal of waste/toxins via the bile and the urine and spares the potassium that is otherwise lost with conventional diuretics. Dandelion is also an excellent herb for erectile dysfunction, orchitis (inflammation of the testes) and urinary tract infections.

Dandelion is a rich source of nutrients like potassium, iron and vitamins A, B, C and D and also contains anti-inflammatory compounds that make it effective in dealing with arthritic pain. It is believed to be effective in dealing with symptoms of arthritis, rheumatism and other chronic joint pain conditions as it is capable of flushing out toxins that cause the joints and muscles to become inflamed. In addition, it can reduce the level of uric acid in the body, which results in reduced pain and stiffness in the joints and increased joint mobility and can help to relieve the symptoms of gout.

Dill *(Anethum graveolens)*

Dill is a tall and easily grown herb that does well in sun or partial shade. The feathery leaves, flowers and seeds have exceptional health benefits and the flavour goes exceedingly well with fish dishes. Dill has unique health benefits from two types of healing components, monoterpenes (carvone, limonene and anethofuran) and flavonoids (kaempferol and vicenin). The monoterpene components can activate the enzyme glutathione-S-transferase, which helps attach the antioxidant molecule, glutathione, to oxidise molecules that would otherwise do damage in the body.

The activity of dill's volatile oils makes it a 'chemo-protective' food, like parsley, that can help neutralise particular types of carcinogens, such as the benzopyrenes that are part of cigarette and charcoal grill smoke. The volatile oils in dill, like garlic, also have bacteria-regulating effects so are helpful for the intestines. In addition, dill is a very good source of calcium, which is important for reducing the bone loss that occurs after menopause and is helpful for other conditions, such as rheumatoid arthritis. It is also a good source of dietary fibre and the minerals manganese, iron and magnesium.

Echinacea *(Echinacea purpurea, Echinacea angustifolia, coneflower)*

Echinacea is one of the easiest members of the daisy family to grow and prefers well-drained soil and a sunny position, but it will tolerate dappled shade. Modern scientific studies now validate echinacea's traditional usage as a topical agent to help the body repair skin wounds and internally to enhance the immune system. The active constituents, which are thought to bolster the body's defence, are known to be polysaccharides that stimulate the activity of macrophages - the white blood cells that destroy bacteria, fungi, viruses, other foreign invaders and even wayward cancerous cells. Echinacea also activates the body's production of interferon, a specific protein which protects cells against the invasion of viruses.

Fennel *(Foeniculum vulgare)*

Fennel is an easy plant to grow but must be kept moist (but not soaked) and the soil must be earthed-up around the bulb as it grows. Both the bulb and the seeds have exceptional properties and have been used for centuries for both culinary and medicinal purposes. In India it is common to chew fennel seeds after meals to facilitate digestion as they help prevent and treat flatulence by expelling gases from the stomach. The oils in fennel seeds have antacid properties and help to facilitate proper absorption of nutrients in the stomach and intestines.

Fennel seeds not only can help prevent and treat constipation but can also act as a laxative with their high-fibre content. They help clear the bowels and their stimulating effect helps maintain the proper peristaltic motion of the intestines. They also help to eliminate worms and parasites. Studies have also shown that fennel may inhibit the formation of certain tumours caused by cancer-causing chemicals as it helps detoxify and remove waste material from the body and protects against ageing and related degenerative diseases.

Fennel seeds can help to improve the vision and hair, relax the body, sharpen the memory and have a cooling effect when one becomes over-heated. Their antioxidant properties make them a powerful anti-inflammatory which inhibits oxidation, thus preventing many chronic conditions that cause fevers and pain when taken as a tea. The following are health issues fennel seeds can improve and help to treat:

- Alzheimer's disease and dementia
- Arthritis
- Cancer
- Colic pain and indigestion for babies
- Colitis
- Constipation
- Cough, cold and sore throats
- Crohn's disease
- Diarrhoea
- Flatulence
- Gastrointestinal disorders

- Glaucoma
- Heart disease
- High blood pressure
- High cholesterol
- Immune system disorders
- Indigestion
- Insomnia
- Lactation problems of nursing mothers
- Liver disorders
- Macular degeneration
- Menstrual problems
- Rheumatism
- Stroke

Ginger *(Gingiber officinalis, Zingiber officinale)*

Ginger can be grown easily indoors or outside from a part of a root (rhizome) and makes a perfect indoor herb to grow in pots. It is very low-maintenance, loves partial sunlight and parts of the root can be used as required leaving the rest to continue growing.

Ginger has antioxidant, antiseptic and expectorant properties, increases energy levels, promotes perspiration in a fever, cleanses the digestive tract in cases of diarrhoea and thins the blood. It also helps the body to eliminate wastes through the skin and acts as a catalyst for other herbs, to increase their effectiveness. The following are health issues ginger can help to treat.

- Bronchitis
- Colds and coughs
- Diarrhoea
- Digestion problems
- *Helicobacter pylori* infection
- High blood pressure
- Influenza
- Morning and motion sickness
- Muscle and menstrual cramps
- Poor circulation
- Sore throat

Consuming 2 grams of ginger per day can produce significantly higher insulin sensitivity, which is beneficial to diabetics, as well as lower LDL ('bad') cholesterol and triglycerides. Ginger can be taken with food or as a tea and the raw peeled root can be dabbed onto the affected area for relief of hives. Externally, ginger can also be applied as a fomentation for the treatment of pain, inflammation and stiff joints. Simmer one ounce of dried ginger root in two quarts of water for 10 minutes. Strain and soak a cloth in the water and apply to the affected area. Keep changing the cloth to keep a constant warm temperature on the skin. The skin should become red as the circulation increases.

For children and adults with bronchial coughs: mix ginger root powder with a non-petroleum jelly and rub on the chest to help loosen coughs and expel mucus.

NOTE: Avoid ginger if taking anticoagulants (blood thinning medication), hormone therapies and contraceptive pills or non-steroidal anti-inflammatory medications, such as aspirin and ibuprofen. Also avoid it with heart problems or during the first three months of pregnancy or if breast feeding.

Lemon balm *(Melissa officinalis,* melissa oil*)*

The name 'Melissa' means honey bee in Greek. Lemon balm is easy to grow and very attractive to bees, giving their honey a lemony scent. This herb was brought to Britain by the Romans and has soothing and sedative properties which help with relaxation and sleep. It is also useful to treat colic, poor digestion, vertigo and vomiting and was often used by Avicenna, the famous Arab physician. It makes a refreshing tea that calms anxiety, restores depleted energy, enhances the memory and acts as a decongestant and antihistamine, helping with problems like asthma or allergies.

Lemon balm leaf tea, with mint or peppermint leaves and a teaspoon of locally produced honey, can eliminate hay fever symptoms and reduce bloating and flatulence. Make the tea as below but include the mint or peppermint leaves, then reheat and add the honey; sip slowly. To make a tea, pour hot water onto a handful of leaves in a jar. Screw on the lid and when cool, leave to chill for four hours in the refrigerator, then serve with ice.

The tea also has antiviral and antibacterial properties so can be used to dab onto spots and other rashes at night to relieve itching and help them to heal faster. The essential oil can be used as an insect and mosquito repellent. Crush a handful of the leaves in the hand and rub them on exposed skin.

NOTE: Sun on the skin must be avoided after applying lemon balm to avoid sunburn.

Lemongrass *(Cymbopogon)*

Lemongrass can easily be grown at home. Take a few stalks and place the bulb end in water and allow to soak until roots form. This may take anywhere from two weeks to a month. Once the lemongrass has developed roots 1.25 to 2.5 centimetres (½ to 1 inch) long, plant in the garden or in a pot with lots of rich soil. Lemongrass likes sun and warm temperatures, so keep it indoors as a houseplant in the winter and place near a south-facing window.

Lemongrass is a tall stalked plant with a lemony scent and provides a zesty lemon flavour and aroma to many Thai dishes. It is known to have numerous health benefits, especially when used in combination with other Thai spices, such as garlic, fresh chillies and coriander. Thailand's favourite soup, *tom yum kung*, is thought to be capable of combating colds, influenza and even some cancers. Lemongrass is also useful for catarrh, colic, congestive and neuralgic forms of dysmenorrhoea, diarrhoea, fever, flatulence, menstruation disorders, muscle spasms and vomiting. For fevers, combine with ginger, honey and cinnamon. It is also beneficial for children's digestive system.

Externally, it can be used to treat athletes foot, chronic rheumatism, lice, lumbago, neuralgia, ringworm, scabies and sprains. Mix with pure coconut oil to apply as a liniment. Citronella oil is derived from the leaves and stems of lemongrass and is an excellent insect repellent, especially against mosquitoes, and can also be used as an effective household cleaner without harsh chemical additives.
NOTE: Lemongrass is extremely fibrous and therefore must be cooked thoroughly. If making a soup, boil the lemongrass for at least 10 minutes in order for it to soften adequately.

Marjoram *(Origanum majorana)*
Marjoram is easy to grow in pots or containers and in the ground. It will die back in the winter but will return the next spring. The seeds are slow to germinate so are best sown indoors at 21°C (70°F). In order to dry marjoram, pick the leaves just after flower buds appear

but before they open, removing no more than a third of the plant's leaves in a single harvest.

A tea made from marjoram can help to relieve an upset stomach, colic, headache, high blood pressure, motion sickness, seasickness and a variety of nervous complaints. It can be used for cramps and nausea associated with menstruation and for other severe cases of abdominal cramps. It can be added to the bath to promote a calming effect and to relieve insomnia. Marjoram can also be applied as a fomentation to painful swellings and rheumatic joints and in salves to stimulate the circulation.

Milk thistle *(Silybum marianum)*
The milk thistle plant grows to about one metre in height, with glossy, veined leaves and five-centimetre purple summer flowers. It is easily maintained and, although it likes full sun and moderate watering, it can also tolerate drought and partial shade. All parts of the milk thistle plant are edible and medicinally the active ingredient, silymarin, found in the seeds, is a powerful protector and can cleanse the liver of many industrial toxins, such as carbon tetrachloride, and more common agents like alcohol.

Mint *(Mentha arvensis)*
Always grow plants of the mint family in a large pot or container as they spread very easily. Once established, mint will die back during the winter and then return each year thereafter and need little attention. Mint leaves soaked in vinegar are especially good when

consumed with peas, potatoes and lamb. Mint is anti-inflammatory, antiseptic, anti-fungal and a stimulant for the heart and circulatory system. It is useful in chills, fevers, coughs, colds, 'flu, hiccups, colic, wind, nausea, diarrhoea, constipation and irritable bowel syndrome. Use externally for skin infections, cuts, grazes and sores and the oil can help to relieve toothache. Mint vapours can be inhaled to relieve the effects of a cold.

Nettles *(Urtica dioica)*
Nettles are prolific and found all over the world. They appear, uninvited, in almost every garden and are probably one of the most well-known and hated plants on the planet. They thrive almost anywhere, lie dormant in the winter and re-grow from underground stems in the spring. They can reach a height of four feet in one season. They are best grown in a container for this reason. It is possible to pick nettles without being stung if they are grasped hard enough to force the stinging hairs flat so that they cannot penetrate the skin, and they lose their stinging ability when dried or cooked.

Nettles are a valuable food source that is rich in protein, vitamins A, B complex and C and minerals such as calcium, potassium, magnesium and iron. The tips of the young leaves are consumed as a nutritious vegetable in France. A tea made from nettle seeds is a remedy against infection caused by animal bites and can act as an antidote to poisoning from hemlock, henbane, mandrake and nightshade plants. A tea made with nettle leaves, dandelion leaves, rosehips and honey has outstanding medicinal properties which can help to remedy all the following health issues.

- Alzheimer's disease
- Anaemia
- Asthma
- Arthritis
- Bladder infections
- Bronchitis
- Bursitis
- Flatulence
- Gingivitis
- Gout
- Kidney or bladder stones
- Hay fever
- Hives
- Laryngitis
- Menstrual problems
- Multiple sclerosis
- Nose polyps
- Pleurisy
- Prostate enlargement
- Sciatica
- Sore throat
- Worms

NOTE: Do not drink nettle tea if suffering from heart problems. Externally, the juice from the leaves or a tea made from the roots can be used as a wash for skin infections and rashes and even gangrene.

Oregano *(Origanum compactum)*

The Greeks described oregano as 'the joy of the mountains' and it has been used for centuries both as an aromatic herb in cooking and for its powerful medicinal properties. It is an easy-to-care-for herb that can be grown in pots inside or outside and in the ground and is favoured in Italian dishes.

Oregano helps to settle flatulence and stimulates the flow of bile.

It is also a useful promoter of menstruation and can relieve headaches. It is often used in the treatment of colds and influenza and an infusion is used to treat coughs, including whooping cough. Oregano can effectively fight food poisoning bacteria, the *Toxoplasmosis gondii* parasite, the norovirus (winter vomiting disease) and the intestinal infection *Helicobacter pylori*. It can also lessen the ageing effect of pollution and help in the treatment of diabetes, reduce cholesterol and protect against cancer.

Oregano contains carvacrol, which is very effective in lowering blood pressure. It reduces the heart rate, mean arterial pressure, and both the diastolic and systolic blood pressures. It is also a viable alternative to salt in meals. A high-sodium diet can lead to high blood pressure as each teaspoon of salt has more than 2300 milligrams of sodium whereas oregano is a sodium-free food. A low-sodium diet for individuals with high blood pressure has a limit of 1500 milligrams per day.

As with basil, it has been suggested that eating plenty of oregano can help repel mosquitos. Oregano has many of the medicinal attributes of the other marjoram herbs, but also contains further essential oils which make it much more antiseptic in action, both internally and externally, and it can be used as an effective mouthwash for inflammation of the mouth and throat.

Externally it is useful for infected cuts and wounds and may be applied as a hot fomentation to relieve painful swellings and rheumatism, as well as for colic. A lotion may be made which will soothe stings and bites.

Making a household cleanser and surface sanitiser using oregano oil or a tea from oregano leaves is especially useful where people may be vulnerable to the effects of strong bleach or alcohol-based cleaners, such as care homes, hospitals and schools.

Parsley *(Petroselinum crispum)*

Parsley can be grown easily both in pots indoors and outdoors and in the ground and has been used medicinally since the time of the Ancient Greeks. Early use was mainly as fodder for horses but eventually it gained a growing reputation as a culinary and medicinal herb.

It is one of the most potent foods of the common vegetable kingdom; as a juice, if properly and completely extracted, it is wise to drink no more than 120 millilitres (four fluid ounces) daily without the addition of other vegetable juices because otherwise it can seriously disturb the nervous system. With the addition of the raw juice of carrots and celery it is very valuable as nourishment for the optic system, also for the kidneys and bladder and as an aid in allaying inflammation of the urethra and genital organs.

Parsley can clear toxins from the body, inhibit tumour growth, relax spasms and reduce inflammation and can be an effective remedy for anaemia, anorexia, arthritis, colic, cramps, dyspepsia, flatulence, fluid retention, indigestion, menstrual complaints, rheumatism and urinary tract problems. It can also induce lactation for women trying to breast feed.

Parsley also stimulates the secretion of digestive juices

and helps considerably in disorders of the kidneys, liver and spleen. When eating meat, finely chopped raw parsley should be eaten at the same time, because of its diuretic action, in order to stimulate the elimination of the excessive uric acid resulting from the digestion of meat. When eaten after a meal it can help to freshen the breath. Parsley can also be used externally, as a tea, on abscesses, eczema, itchy skin, rashes, toothache and wounds and it kills head lice.

NOTE: Parsley is not suitable for medicinal use by pregnant women.

Peppermint *(Mentha piperita)*

As with mint (see page 95), peppermint is best grown in a container or pot and is suitable for indoors or outdoors. First described in England in 1696, peppermint and its oil have been used in Eastern and Western traditional medicine for treating cancer, colds, cramps, indigestion, infections, nausea, sore throat, toothache and worms and parasites. Today, the oil is used widely as a flavouring for chewing gum, toothpaste, mouthwash, cigarettes and drugs.

It is also used as an ingredient in cough and cold preparations and for irritable bowel syndrome (IBS) and the menthol it contains is used in many antiseptic, anti-itch and local anaesthetic preparations. Peppermint has astringent properties and can calm the stomach, intestinal tract and nervous system. It also stimulates menstrual flow and the salivary glands to help with digestion and can help to fight off bacterial infections. Peppermint oil can also effectively repel ants, mice and rats as they cannot stand the aroma.

NOTE: Avoid peppermint oil if pregnant or suffering from gastric reflux or active stomach ulcers and do not apply peppermint oil to the face, especially under the nose of a child or infant.

Rosemary *(Rosmarinus officinalis)*

Rosemary is an exceptionally easy plant to grow indoors or outside in pots and containers or the ground. It will withstand harsh winters and provide its stems and leaves for use all year round. It is especially good with red meats like rabbit and venison.

Rosemary has antibacterial, antifungal, anti-inflammatory, antioxidant and antiseptic properties, stimulates the circulation and detoxifies the system. It is useful for treating a poor memory and poor concentration and is used for a wide range of other conditions, such as circulatory problems, colds, coughs, diabetes, flatulence, influenza, nervous complaints and stomach cramps and as a mild stimulant.

It can also fight food poisoning bacteria, lessen the ageing effect of pollution and protect against cancer. Rosemary tea is useful for treating *Candida* infections and as a mouthwash for sore gums and a gargle for sore throats. It is also commonly used as an aspirin substitute for headaches and can improve digestion.

Externally, the diluted essential oil is also a warming ingredient in ointment for aches, painful joints, muscle stiffness and rheumatism. It can also be used as a tonic for the hair and scalp in shampoos or hair lotions as it increases circulation and scalp stimulation and can combat dandruff and has been said even to help to prevent baldness.

Neem leaves, rosemary and lavender contain natural insecticidal properties and act as an antiseptic. These herbs together with aroma therapeutic ingredients, such as tea tree oil and rose geranium, have the ability to eliminate external parasites, including pubic lice, and prevent re-infestation, and can be used as a toxin-free household cleaner. Greek fishermen cover their catch with rosemary to prevent spoilage.

NOTE: Avoid rosemary if pregnant or breastfeeding or suffering from high blood pressure.

Sage *(Salvia officinalis)*

Sage is an easy-to-grow pot herb known, since Ancient Roman times, as the guardian over all other herbs and has been in use in various traditional European and Chinese medicines for its health-promoting and disease-preventing properties. It has anti-allergic, antifungal, anti-inflammatory and antiseptic properties and helps check excessive mucus in the body.

Sage is good for treating anxiety, depression, excessive salivation, female sterility, indigestion, flatulence, profuse perspiration and night sweats (especially menopausal) and can reduce excessive lactation in breastfeeding mothers. It should not be used for more than a week, but during this period, the tea may be taken up to three times per day. Externally it is good for treating acne, gum, mouth and throat infections, insect bites and vaginal discharge and combats oily hair and scalp.

NOTE: Sage should be avoided if pregnant or suffering from epilepsy.

Tarragon *(Artemisia dranunculus)*

Tarragon is an easily grown age-old herb that should be harvested regularly. Three plants should be enough to provide sufficient for both culinary and medicinal use. Like dill, it is a good herb to accompany eggs, fish and seafood dishes. Medicinally, tarragon can fight food poisoning bacteria and inhibit the growth of *Helicobacter pylori* in the intestines. It also lessens the ageing effect of pollution, helps in the treatment of diabetes, reduces cholesterol and blood pressure and protects against cancer.

Thyme and lemon thyme *(Thymus vulgaris, Thymus citriodorus)*

Thyme is a slow-growing evergreen herb that will be happy in pots and containers or in the ground. A tea made with thyme is commonly used for bronchial problems, such as acute bronchitis, whooping cough and laryngitis and is also beneficial for the treatment of diarrhoea, gastritis and lack of appetite. It can also help to treat alcoholism, excess mucus, hangovers, headaches, parasites and worms, respiratory problems and stomach problems, including cramps. It is said that thyme is to the trachea and bronchitis what peppermint is to the intestines and stomach. It contains an aromatic oil called thymol that is responsible for many of its excellent properties.

Externally, its antiseptic properties make it a useful mouthwash and cleansing wash for the skin. It will destroy fungal infections such as athlete's foot and skin parasites such as crabs, lice and scabies. For those purposes, a tincture should be made from 115 grams (four ounces) of dried thyme to a pint of alcohol. (For guidance on how to make a tincture, see www.naturecures.co.uk and the comprehensive *Nature Cures – the A to Z of Ailments and Natural Foods*.

Fruit

Growing fruit bushes and trees can be very rewarding when harvest time arrives. There are now many miniature species of fruit trees available that can be grown in pots in small spaces and provide a harvest far quicker than the larger, older varieties. Some small fruits, such as berries, will need protecting from birds who will often steal them before you have noticed they are ready for picking.

Apples *(Malus domestica)*

According to scientific research, the old saying, 'An apple a day keeps the doctor away' is actually a fact, not just folklore. Apple skin is a major source of a potent flavonoid called quercetin and regular consumption can help to prevent breast cancer. Another flavonoid, found only in apples, called phloridzin, can help prevent bone loss associated with menopause.

Apples are found to be most consistently associated with a reduced risk of asthma, cancer, heart disease and type 2 diabetes when compared with other fruits and vegetables. In addition, eating apples is also associated with increased lung function and weight loss. They are even said to help combat cholera. Apples work in a dose-dependent manner, meaning the more apples are eaten, the greater the protection.

Avocado *(Persea americana)*

Avocados can be easily grown from the stone in the fruit. Firstly, remove the stone carefully (without cutting it) and then wash it clean of all the flesh (often it helps to soak it in water for a few minutes and then scrub all the remaining fruit off). Be careful not to remove the brown skin as that is the seed cover. Then, with the pointed end facing upwards, take four toothpicks and stick them at a slight downward angle into the avocado stone, spaced evenly around its circumference. Then stand the avocado in a clear glass of water that comes up to the sticks (about half way up the stone) and stand on a sunny windowsill. Change the water daily and make sure to keep it topped up, especially when roots have begun to emerge.

When a sprout has appeared and grown to about 15-18 centimetres (6-7 inches) high, cut it back to about 8 centimetres (3 inches), leaving two or three leaves, and this will encourage new growth. When it reaches 15-18 centimetres (6-7 inches) again, pot it up in a rich humus soil, leaving the top half of the stone exposed, and place on a sunny windowsill. Keep turning the plant to ensure it grows up straight.

Components in avocados can contribute towards the prevention of heart disease, boost the immune system in the elderly and improve male fertility. Avocado may be high in fat, but most of it is the healthy monounsaturated type which is essential for plump, youthful skin and actually helps neutralise the 'bad' fat in other foods, meaning it could help with weight loss. Avocado lowers LDL cholesterol and is a good source of potassium, which helps the body flush out toxins. It also contains the most potent anti-ageing combination, vitamin E and vitamin C, which mop up ageing free radicals and de-clog arteries. It also contains vitamins K and B6 and fibre.

Berries and currants

Berries and currants (black, red, white) do not take up as much space as fruit trees and can be trained against a wall or fence, and some, like strawberries, can be grown in hanging baskets. They will need some protection from birds who will steal the fruits the minute they have ripened. All berries and currants help to prevent varicose veins, ease rheumatoid arthritis, reduce the risks of cancer and have antibacterial properties. Berries and currants are rich in vitamins C, K and B9, fibre and many powerful phytonutrients. They all help the body make collagen, the protein needed to keep skin supple, smooth and healthy. Dark-coloured berries contain potent anthocyanins that are antioxidants that help the body cleanse itself of free radicals (see page 21).

Bilberries are known to improve eyesight, especially night vision. Blackcurrants protect against UV skin damage and reduce the ageing effect of sunburn by neutralising free radicals. Cranberries and blueberries both help protect against cystitis by stopping harmful bacteria stick to the lining of the urinary tract. Strawberries are particularly good for respiratory conditions and can help to protect smoker's lungs from damage.

Cherries *(Prunus avium, Prunus cerasus, Malpighia emarginata)*

Cherry trees can be grown as dwarf versions for smaller spaces and provide plenty of fruit in the autumn. Cherries are very rich in melatonin, the 'sleep hormone' that can cross the blood-brain barrier easily and produces soothing effects on the brain neurons, calming down nervous system irritability and helping to relieve anxiety, headaches, insomnia and neurosis. The acerola cherry has the highest content of vitamin C of all fruits and the morello or Brazilian sour cherry has powerful anti-inflammatory and pain-relieving properties.

NOTE: Cherry stones are toxic. If a cherry pip is chewed, crushed or somehow damaged, it automatically produces hydrogen cyanide. Symptoms of mild poisoning include anxiety, confusion, dizziness, headache and vomiting. Larger doses can lead to difficulty breathing, increased blood pressure and heart rate and kidney failure, and reactions can include coma, convulsions and death from respiratory arrest.

Citrus fruits *(Lemons Citrus limonum, Limes Citrus aurantifolia Oranges Citrus aurantium Tangerines Citrus tangerina)*

Dwarf lemon, lime, orange and tangerine trees can be grown in large pots and brought inside during the winter; all citrus fruits are exceptionally good to grow health wise. They provide protection against oesophageal, oropharyngeal/laryngeal (mouth, larynx and pharynx) and stomach cancers.

Lemon juice can act as an anti-acid for digestive problems and is antibacterial, antifungal, antiseptic, antiviral and a cleanser of blood, liver, lymph glands and kidneys and a natural diuretic. It is also good for treating acne, constipation, heartburn, hiccups, nausea, respiratory ailments, parasites and worms, and thrush.

Lemon is one of the very low glycaemic fruits (it does not raise blood sugar) so is also good for diabetics and the citric acid in lemons can help to dissolve bladder and kidney stones. The abundance of phyto-chemical antioxidants and soluble, as well as insoluble, dietary fibre, is helpful in reducing the risk of cancer and many chronic diseases, such as arthritis, obesity and coronary heart disease.

Lemon also helps to regulate blood pressure and can alleviate depression, stress and anxiety. Its juice is more effective in healing oral thrush in HIV patients than the standard remedy of gentian violet. Traditionally, lemon peel oil has been used to discourage intestinal parasites, while the vitamin C-rich juice and rind help to increase bone mineral density. The consumption of one lemon per day (including half of the rind and pith) can provide protection against all the above ailments and can be added to teas for additional benefits as well as fish and vegetable dishes.

Limes have many of the attributes of lemons but also have powerful antibacterial properties that can prevent infection from the *Vibrio cholera* bacteria. They can also reduce cholesterol levels and prevent scurvy and have been known to help smokers recover from the damage caused and cravings for nicotine.

Nobiletin and **tangeretin**, found in orange and tangerine peel, can lower cholesterol more effectively than some prescription drugs and without side effects. Grating a tablespoon or so of the peel from a well-scrubbed tangerine or orange each day and using it to flavour tea, salads, salad dressings, yoghurt, soups, or hot oatmeal, buckwheat or rice, is a good way of naturally lowering cholesterol levels. Both of these flavonoids can also function as blood thinners and are anti-inflammatory, and with the added benefit of vitamin C, oranges and tangerines may help prevent heart attacks and strokes. Tangerines can also help with weight loss as they contain compounds that stimulate fat burning.

Figs *(Ficus carica)*

Figs grow well in large containers that are on pot stands to allow drainage or in the ground in a sunny position near a wall for wind protection. Traditionally their roots have been restricted as this is thought to increase fruit production.

Figs promote good sleeping habits and therefore can help to prevent insomnia. They increase energy, promote stronger bones and are helpful in treating constipation due to their laxative effect. They also have an analgesic effect against insect stings and bites. The fruit is also given as a cure for piles and diarrhoea and lessens the acid in the stomach, which can be helpful to pregnant women. Figs are also said to increase sexual desire and promote overall longevity and good health.

Fig leaves are best known for treating diabetes, but there

are many other uses, such as remedying boils, bronchitis, cancer, cardiovascular disease, fungal infections, genital warts, liver cirrhosis, haemorrhoids, high blood pressure, ringworm, shingles, skin problems and ulcers. Diabetics need less insulin when they regularly consume fig leaf extract. They should take the extract with breakfast, first thing in the morning. An additional remedy is to boil the leaves of the fig in some freshly filtered or bottled mineral water and drink this as a tea. Other medicinal uses are as follows:

- Cardiovascular and cancer patients should drink fig leaf tea and eat two fresh figs daily.
- Genital warts: Take one fig leaf and apply the sap from the leaf to the affected areas.
- Haemorrhoids: Place three leaves in one litre of water and boil for at least 15 minutes. Remove from the heat and let it cool. Remove the leaves from the tea and use as a bath or apply to the affected areas.
- Hair and scalp: Use fig leaves as a decoction to condition hair and treat fungal infections of the scalp.
- Liver cirrhosis: Take four fig leaves, wash and pound them. Fill a glass with water (preferably bottled mineral water), add the leaves and drink this twice a day.
- High blood pressure: Place three fig leaves in half a litre of water. Boil for 15 minutes and drink daily.
- Ringworm: Cut open a leaf and take the sap. Rub on the ringworm. This remedy works very quickly for ringworm as well as boils, fungal infections and warts.

- Shingles: Place four fig leaves in one litre of water. Boil for a few minutes, allow to cool and remove the leaves. Take a wash cloth, dip it in the water and apply to the affected area.
- Skin disorders: If the leaves are mashed, they can be used as a skin cleanser for acne and pimples, as can fig leaf tea.
- Stomach and mouth ulcers: Every day chew two fig leaves and swallow the whole leaf. People with advanced ulcers should do this in the morning on an empty stomach.

Grapes *(Vitis vinifera)*

Grapes require a long and frost-free growing season and need to be supported by a trellis or pergola. They will not produce fruit until the third year so patience is needed. Because it is now so rare to find grapes with seeds in the supermarket, it can be beneficial to grow some as there are compounds in the seeds that can help to prevent cancer, diabetes and neurodegenerative diseases such as Parkinson's and Alzheimer's disease.

Scientific studies have also shown that there are inorganic mineral compounds, such as iridium and rhodium, in grape seeds, and colloidal gold in black grape skins. These compounds cause cancer cells to 'commit suicide' within 24 hours, without damaging surrounding cells, due to their ability to activate a protein called JNK (c-Jun N-terminal kinase) that regulates apoptosis (cell suicide).

All grapes contain compounds that strengthen the capillaries and protect against thread veins and skin sagging, but red and black grape skins also contain 20 known antioxidants that work together to fend off the free radical attacks that lead to disease. Grapes can cleanse the blood and help with recovery from injury and infection, which is why they became a traditional gift for people who were unwell.

Kiwi fruit *(Actinidia deliciosa, Actinidia chinensis,* Chinese gooseberry, yang toa*)*

Kiwi fruit plants are vines that can be grown against a fence or wall or over a pergola or archway. Tie in new shoots as they grow to give them support. If growing just one kiwi fruit bush, ensure it is a self-fertile variety as the female plant produces the fruit and the male plant is required for pollination. Always protect young shoots from frost with a fleece and harvest before any frost appears. Unripe kiwi fruit can be kept in the bottom of a refrigerator for three or four months. To hasten ripening place them in a fruit bowl at room temperature with bananas.

Kiwi fruit can reduce the risk of cancer and detoxify the blood. They can also reduce wheezing, chronic coughing and mucus production, especially in children suffering from asthma and other respiratory disorders. Kiwis are a rich source of the antioxidant chlorophyll and of vitamin C (even more than oranges) and vitamin K and a good source of vitamin E, copper and fibre. Kiwis contain as much potassium as bananas and the seeds contain omega-3 fatty acids. They are also a good source of magnesium and phosphorus. Always consume the skin as this provides triple the amount of fibre and vitamin C.

Pears *(Pyrus communis)*
Pear trees do need a lot of space as they can grow to 12 metres (40 feet) in height unless pruned annually, but pears are a nutritious and low-calorie fruit which have many health benefits. Pear skins are rich in copper, fibre and chlorogenic acid. All these compounds can help to lower cholesterol levels and prevent colon disorders, thereby reducing the risk of irritable bowel syndrome and colon cancer from developing.

Pears are often recommended by healthcare practitioners as a hypoallergenic fruit that is less likely to produce an adverse response than other fruits and they are particularly useful as the introductory fruit when weaning infants.

Flowers

Many types of flowers can be helpful to grow alongside vegetables to attract beneficial insects and repel garden pests, as mentioned above. Marigolds and nasturtiums are especially useful in this regard and are very easy to grow from seed. The following three are also edible and have exceptional medicinal benefits.

Marigold *(Calendula officinalis)*
Marigold is often used in lotions or ointments as a natural antiseptic and to aid wound healing and prevent wound infection, for burns, sores, abrasions, wind burn, fungal skin infections and varicose veins. It can also be used as a mouth wash after tooth extraction

and for inflamed gums and laryngitis. Extracts can be taken internally to cure inflammation of the stomach or gall bladder and to aid healing after surgery. A tea can be made to expel worms and parasites that will also heal any tissue damage the worms have caused in the bowels.

Nasturtium *(Tropaeolum majus)*

Nasturtiums are one of the easiest plants to grow and will climb and spread around the plants that they can help to protect from aphids. The leaves, seeds and flowers have been used medicinally for centuries. The leaves are an appetite stimulant, antiscorbutic (prevents or cures scurvy), depurative (cleanses wastes and toxins from the body), diuretic, expectorant, purgative (improves bowel action), hypoglycaemic, odontalgic (relieves toothache), stimulant and stomachic (improves digestion).

Nasturtium's peppery leaves and flowers are rich in vitamin C, while the seeds are high in iron. The flowers can be used as a colourful and nutritious culinary garnish and flowers and leaves can be steeped in hot water to make a tea. The freshly pressed juice has been used internally and externally in the treatment of the ailments listed below.

- Bronchitis
- Digestive disorders
- Hair disorders
- Hyperthyroidism
- Influenza
- Kidney disorders
- Odontalgia (toothache)
- Respiratory disorders
- Scurvy
- Skin disorders

- Tuberculosis
- Urinary tract infection
- Water retention

Nasturtium leaves or petals can be ground up using a mortar and pestle to make a paste that has antibiotic, antiseptic and antifungal properties and can be used to treat acne, minor cuts and skin irritation and as an effective hair tonic, helping to promote the growth of thick hair.

Sunflowers *(Helianthus annus)*

The sunflower's name comes from the Greek 'helios', meaning sun and 'anthos', meaning flower and 'annus' meaning annual. According to Linnaeus, they were the only flowering plant known to him that lived for a single season. Sunflowers are very easy and enjoyable to grow but need plenty of sunshine and water as they are vigorous plants and some species can grow up to a height of 4 metres (10 or 12 feet). The large heads provide hundreds of nutritious seeds and the flowers are very attractive to bees.

There are powerful components in sunflower oil and the seeds that can reduce cholesterol and protect against heart disease. They can also slow down the ageing process and help to fight infection and inflammatory skin diseases. The seeds and oil of the sunflower are very rich sources of omega-3 fatty acids, copper, magnesium, manganese, phosphorus, selenium, and vitamins B1, B3, B6, B9 and E.

Feeding your health-garden plants

The condition of your soil and feeding your plants are important in order to gain the most nutrients. These nutrients come out of complex organic matter as soil bacteria break it down and are then taken up by the plants.

Ash

Using the ash from a wood-burning stove or having a wood-burning bin in the garden is very useful because the ash from wood can contain many useful nutrients for your food crops, such as calcium carbonate, copper, iron, magnesium, phosphate, potash and zinc. The amount of each will vary depending on the type of wood burnt.

The calcium carbonate in wood ash is very alkaline (meaning it has a high pH), so ashes can be used as an effective liming agent to raise the pH levels in acidic soils. Wood ash is water-soluble, which means it can spread through soil instantly and have an immediate effect on the soil's pH levels. However, it should never be used where seedlings are to be planted.

Ash is also very useful to add to the compost bin as the worms, that will be working very hard to create the soil, thrive better in an alkaline environment. Plants that like an alkaline soil are:

- Asparagus
- Juniper
- California lilacs
- Currants
- Forsythia
- Gooseberries
- Mock oranges
- Spirea
- Hellebores
- Clematis
- Dianthus
- Asian persimmon
- Lavender
- Parsley
- Okra

Ash should never be given as a feed or mulch around acid-preferring crops such as:

- Blueberries
- Rhododendrons
- Potatoes and most other annual vegetables.

NOTE: It is very important to keep the ashes dry when storing as potassium is easily washed out.

Chicken pellets

Chicken pellets have a high-nitrogen content and are a good all-round soil improver. Fresh chicken manure must only be added to a compost heap whilst the dried and heat-treated pellets can be added to the soil around most fruits and vegetables, especially leafy crops like cabbage and spinach, salad crops like celery as well as courgettes, fruit bushes, rhubarb, potatoes and sweet corn.

Comfrey

Comfrey roots gather potassium from the soil and collect it in the leaves. It is therefore worth growing a patch of comfrey, harvesting the leaves of a few plants and mulching around any fruit or rose bushes. Adding comfrey to the compost bin can also help to provide extra potassium. Soaking some comfrey leaves in a bucket of water for a week can provide a good feed for potatoes that need potassium.

Compost

It is always a good idea to have your own compost bin, if there is space, to which you can add your organic cuttings and weeds etc. You can also add your kitchen scraps but never put any cooked vegetables or animal products in it as this will attract unwanted vermin into your garden. Egg shells can be added for extra calcium but make sure they are washed well first. Compost helps to provide extra nutrients for your food crops when it is dug into the soil and left for a few weeks before planting seeds or seedlings.

Epsom salts

Add one teaspoon of Epsom salts to four cups of warm water to dissolve it. Then when cool pour into a spray bottle. Use this to spray peppers, roses and tomatoes once, then again 10 days later, to produce more flowers and fruits due to the magnesium content.

Fish, blood and bone meal

Blood provides nitrogen and does not take long to break down. Fish meal provides nitrogen, phosphorus and potassium and bone meal provides mainly phosphorus with some nitrogen and calcium. It is a good all round fertiliser for fruit bushes and trees, herbs and vegetables and should be added to the soil early in the year before plants become vigorous with leaf growth.

Manure

All types of animal, and even human, faeces are excellent soil improvers as the soil microbes break them down and release the nutrients which then feed the plants. However, it is important to use only manure that comes from organically reared animals as the antibiotics and other chemicals used in farming can be absorbed by plants and then consumed by humans. Horse manure is the best type to use. Fresh manure must be rotted in a compost heap for 12 months before being used on plants. Well-rotted manure can be used to improve the soil before planting and as a mulch after plants are established.

Seaweed and kelp

Seaweed and kelp are a very useful fertiliser for mulching plants as they also deter aphids, slugs and snails as well as greatly improving the soil's nutrients. It is always best to keep mulch away from direct contact with the stems of plants. Soaking seaweed or kelp (with a weight to keep it below the water level) then using the resulting thick dark liquid, diluted 20 to one, to feed your plants once a fortnight is another way to provide the nutrients required for a satisfactory harvest. This liquid can also be used as a foliage feed which will also keep garden pests at bay.

Water

Rain water is always best to use for vegetation as it contains many of the nutrients plants require and saves money on water bills; it is therefore a good idea to install water butts on all available drainpipes. Installing an irrigation system is also an economical way to water plants as it can work on a timer at night and a humidity sensor can control it and it can also be connected to water butts. This means that plants will always have all the water they need with no effort required.

Drip feeds on the soil are the best way to water your food crops as spraying water loses much to evaporation and can burn the leaves of plants if done during hot sunshine. Also most of the water will evaporate before it gets a chance to seep down to the roots of plants. Large plants can have a funnel (or a plastic bottle cut in half with the lid off) inserted in the soil near to their roots where water can be poured directly into it, thereby soaking the soil deep down where the roots reside.

Growing food in pots indoors

Most herbs can be grown easily in pots inside the home for use all year round. There are also miniature versions of some fruit bushes, such as lemons and oranges, that can also be grown indoors. Edible houseplants are a wise choice because this is a way to save money while ensuring that these foods are organic and untainted by the chemical sprays so often used on commercially grown food crops. House plants can also help to purify the air in the home which can be polluted by various chemicals that can adversely affect the health.

One example of a very useful medicinal house plant is the aloe vera (*Aloe barbadensis*) which has been known historically for assisting the functions of the gastrointestinal tract and for its properties of soothing, cleansing and helping the body to maintain healthy tissues. Components in this plant, such as acemannan, can aid digestion and blood and lymphatic circulation as well as help to treat asthma, cystic fibrosis, diabetes, epilepsy, irritable bowel syndrome, kidney disorders, liver and gall bladder dysfunction, osteoarthritis and stomach ulcers.

It can also be used externally as an effective treatment for acne, insect bites, sunburn and other skin conditions.

Growing sprouts on your windowsill

Sprouting is a way of reducing the phytic acid levels in legumes, nuts, seeds and grains. Phytic acid is an enzyme inhibitor and reduces the human body's absorption of important minerals such as calcium, copper, iron, magnesium and especially zinc by binding with them in the intestinal tract.

Considered a wonder food, sprouting greens are one of the freshest and most nutritious of all foods available to the human diet. By a process of natural transmutation, sprouted food is easier to digest and has superior nutritional properties when compared with the non-sprouted seed (embryo) from which it emerged.

Sprouted foods have been part of the diet of many ancient races for thousands of years. Even to this day, the Chinese are well known for their mung bean sprouts. Sprouting is so easy and provides a micro-diet of all the essential phytonutrients, vitamins and minerals without the need to consume large quantities of food. They should form a vital component of everyone's diet, especially those trying to recover from any ailments and, as shown below, sprouting requires no soil or constant care except the daily rinsing of water.

Sprouts are good sources of many phytonutrients plus protein, fibre, starch, vitamin A, vitamin B1 (thiamine), vitamin B2 (riboflavin), vitamin B3 (niacin), vitamin B6 (pyridoxine), vitamin B9 (folate), vitamin C, vitamin E and vitamin K. Barley sprouts are also a good source of vitamin B12, which is unusual for plant food sources. They are also good sources of calcium, copper, iron, magnesium, manganese, phosphorus, potassium, selenium, sodium and zinc.

What can be sprouted?

Only choose organic seeds, legumes, grains and nuts and make sure they are for sprouting as seeds produced for growing are often 'dressed', which means they have been coated in fungicidal and antimicrobial substances which are not fit for human consumption.

- **Grains**: Barley, buckwheat, corn, kamut, oat, rice, rye, quinoa and wheat.
- **Legumes**: Chickpea, lentils, mung beans, peas and peanuts.
- **Nuts**: Almonds and hazelnuts.
- **Seeds**: Alfalfa, amaranth, broccoli, cabbage, clover, daikon, fenugreek, flaxseeds, hemp, leek, lemon grass, lettuce, milk thistle, mizuna, mustard, onion, radish, rocket, salba, sesame, spinach, spring onions, sunflower, tatsoi, turnip and watercress.

NOTE: Although whole oats can be sprouted, oat groats sold in food stores which are hulled and require steaming or roasting to prevent rancidity, will not sprout. Whole oats may have an indigestible hull which makes them difficult or even unfit for human consumption.

How are seeds sprouted?

All you need is a small handful of organic seeds, legumes, grains or nuts, one large jam jar, a piece of an old stocking, pair of tights, muslin or other very thin and porous material (enough to cover the jam jar top) and an elastic band or piece of string to secure it.

1. Place the seeds in the jar. They should fill no more than about a tenth of it.
2. Cover with the piece of material and secure with the elastic band or a piece of string.
3. Pour cold water through the material (enough to cover the seeds) shake gently, then tip all of the water back out; otherwise the seeds will just rot. Leave to drain at a 45-degree angle for at least an hour afterwards.
4. Repeat this once or twice a day (making sure you shake the jar so all seeds get well watered) and keep the jar on a window sill.
5. Once the jar is filled with sprouts it is ready for harvesting. This can take around five days or so. When they have filled the jar, either eat them or place them in the refrigerator to slow down growth.

To use, simply take a handful of the sprouts and shake off the seed hulls. It does not matter if some are left as they are not harmful and act as extra fibre, but some may taste a little bitter. The sprouts can be added to salads and sandwiches or as a side dish with meals.

If there are a lot of seeds left, that have not sprouted, it may be because they have not been drained well after rinsing. Make sure to shake the jar and rest it at a 45-degree angle for at least an hour afterwards.

NOTE: During hot weather, mould may grow on the seeds so using a small canvas or muslin bag instead of a jam jar may be more useful. Place the seeds in the bag, then dip it into clean water, shake gently and then hang up to drip dry, repeating this once or twice a day depending on how warm it is. Many people mistake the fine root hairs on sprouts for mould but mould will not appear if:

- The seeds are no older than 12 months and organic.
- The above method is followed and they are rinsed regularly and drained well.
- The container is regularly sterilised between sowings.
- The covering is washed well or changed between sowings.
- The place they are being grown in is not too humid and hot.

Sprouts are an inexpensive, easy and highly nutritious food crop and, because you have grown it yourself, you know it is organic.

Plants that are poisonous to pets and young children

Certain plants should be avoided in the home and garden, if there are animals or young children around, as they are poisonous. Alternatively, they can be grown at a height in a raised bed or hanging basket where animals and young children cannot reach them. It is very rare that a cat or dog will eat plants but sometimes, if they have an upset digestive system, it is a natural instinct for them to chew on some grass or leaves to make themselves vomit. It would be unfortunate if the plant they chose was severely toxic to them, which is why they are all listed here. Houseplants are included as some people put theirs out on a sunny patio, during the summer, within easy reach of children and pets.

- **Amaryllis** (*Amaryllis belladonna, Amaryllis paradisicola*): Ingestion of the many toxins in this popular flowering houseplant can lead to abdominal pain, accelerated defecation, anorexia, dark brown urine, diarrhoea, excessive drooling, gastroenteritis, lethargy, shivering, vomiting and possible contact dermatitis to the mouth, throat, nose and face. Ingestion of larger amounts can cause paralysis, central nervous system collapse and death.

- **Autumn crocus** (*Colchicum autumnale*): contains compounds that attack rapidly dividing cells in the body. Ingestion by animals can cause vomiting, diarrhoea and possible death. It should not be confused with the spring flowering crocuses such as *Crocus chrysanthus, Crocus speciosusas* or *Crocus vernus* as these are not toxic.
- **Azaleas** (*Rhodendron tsutsusi* or *Rhododendron pentanthera*) contain grayanotoxins which can lead to vomiting, seizures and cardiac arrest in all animal species.
- **Avocado** (*Persea americana*) can cause diarrhoea and vomiting in cats and dogs.
- **Bay leaves or laurels** (*Laurus nobilis*) contain grayanotoxins which can lead to vomiting, seizures and cardiac arrest in all animal species.
- **Cannabis** (*Cannabis sativa*) Both the cannabis plant and smoke are toxic to animals and can cause paranoia leading to agitation, anxiety and panting in pets. They may also lose the ability to consume food and water and become dehydrated, which can lead to kidney disorders. Extreme responses to noises, movements and other forms of sensory stimulation may occur. These responses can manifest as trembling or jerking of the head or extremities. In severe cases, the responses may appear similar to seizures.

- **Castor beans** (Ricinus Communis) contain ricin which can cause multiple organ failure in both animals and humans. It is most highly concentrated in the seeds but the seed coating must be damaged to release this toxin; therefore, if seeds are swallowed whole, they may pass through the digestive system and not harm the animal.
- **Cherries** (*Prunus avium, Prunus cerasus*) can cause increased heart rate, rapid breathing, shock and even be fatal in dogs.
- **Chives** (*Allium schoenoprasum*), **garlic** (*Allium sativum*), **leeks** (*Allium ampeloprasum*) , **onions** (*Allium cepa*) and **spring onions** (*Allium fistulosum*) and all other plants in the *Allium* group can cause anaemia and gastrointestinal disorders in cats and dogs.
- **Cyclamen** (*Cyclamen persicum*) is a common houseplant that contains irritating saponins and, when any parts of the plant (especially the tubers or roots) are chewed or ingested by dogs and cats, it can result in clinical signs of drooling, vomiting and diarrhoea. With large ingestions, these plants can result in cardiac problems (abnormal heart rate and rhythm), seizures and death.
- **Bluebell** (*Hyacinthoides non-scripta*), **daffodil** (Narcissus), **hyacinth** (*Hyacinthus*) or **tulip** (*Tulipa*) **bulbs**. When the plant parts or bulbs are chewed or ingested, it can result in tissue irritation to the mouth and oesophagus. Typical signs include profuse drooling, vomiting or diarrhoea. With large ingestions, more severe symptoms, such as an increase in

heart rate, changes in respiration and difficulty breathing, may be seen.
- **Dragon tree** (*Dracaena marginata*) This common houseplant is toxic to dogs and cats.
- **English ivy** (*Hedera helix*) contains many toxins and the cell sap can cause redness, itching and/or blisters when it comes in contact with living tissue. Symptoms include a burning sensation in the throat and mouth followed by redness, blisters, rash, excessive drooling, obvious pain or discomfort of the mouth, pawing at the mouth, hoarseness or weak-sounding vocalisation; excessive desire to drink; gastrointestinal upset, vomiting, diarrhoea and abdominal pain. In cases of an extremely large ingestion: stupor, loss of coordination, hypotension, tachycardia, convulsions and coma can occur.
- **Foxgloves** (*Digitalis purpurae*) contain glycosides which slow down the heart beat and can even stop it and are toxic to all animals.
- **Fruit seeds, cores, stems and stones** from many fruits contain cyanide, which can lead to dilated pupils, difficulty breathing and shock in dogs.
- **Grapes, raisins and currants**, even in small amounts, can cause kidney failure in dogs.
- **Heart leaf philodendron** (*Philodendron oxycardium, Philodendron selloum*) is a common houseplant that is toxic to both animals and children.

- **Hops** (*Humulus Lupulis*), used in beer brewing, can cause a dog's body temperature to rapidly rise to as much as 108° and kill them. Signs are agitation and panting and can be seen within hours of ingestion.
- **Japanese pieris** (*Pieris japonica*) contains grayanotoxins, which can lead to vomiting, seizures and cardiac arrest in all animal species.
- **Japanese yew** (*Taxus cuspidate*) contains compounds that have a direct action upon the heart. Ingestion of any part of the plant (except the fruits) can cause irregular heart beat and even stop the heart, causing death within a few hours in any animal species.
- **Jimson weed** (*Datura stramonium*, Devil's trumpet), can cause restlessness, drunken walking and respiratory failure in cats and dogs.
- **Kalanchoe** (*Bryophyllum pinnatum, Kalanchoe pinnatum*) contains glycosides which slow down the heart beat and can even stop it and be fatal to all animals.
- **Lilies** (*Lilium* – Asiatic, day, Easter, Japanese and tiger varieties) can cause kidney failure in cats.
- **Lily of the valley** (*Convallaria majalis*) contains glycosides, which slow down the heart beat and can even stop it and can be fatal to all animals.
- **Mushrooms** (*Agaricus*) Wild mushrooms can cause vomiting, hallucinations, liver failure and death in dogs.
- **Oleander** (*Nerium oleander*) contains glycosides, which slow

down the heart beat and can even stop it and can be fatal to all animals.
- **Potatoes** (*Solanum tuberosum*) Raw potatoes contain solanine which can cause drooling, vomiting, diarrhoea and severe stomach upset in cats and dogs.
- **Pothos** (*Epipremnum aureum*, devil's ivy, golden pothos): Both the stem and the leaves contain calcium oxalates. Chewing or biting into the plant releases the crystals which penetrate the body's tissues, resulting in injury. It can cause tissue irritation and possible swelling when chewed and lead to oral irritation, intense burning and irritation of mouth, tongue and lips, excessive drooling and foaming at the mouth, difficulty breathing and swallowing, lack of appetite and vomiting.
- **Rhubarb** (*Rheum rhabarbarum*) can cause tremors and kidney failure in cats and dogs. It contains soluble oxalate salts which are absorbed from the gastrointestinal tract and then bind with the body's calcium, resulting in a sudden drop in calcium levels. Rarely, acute renal failure can occur. Clinical signs include drooling, lack of appetite, vomiting, diarrhoea, lethargy, weakness, tremors, bloody urine and changes in thirst and urination in cats and dogs.
- **Sago palm plant** (*Cycas revolute*) can cause diarrhoea, vomiting and seizures in cats and dogs and liver failure in dogs.
- **Shamrock** (*Oxalis triangularis*, sorrel): Rarely, acute renal

failure can occur and other signs are drooling, lack of appetite, vomiting, diarrhoea, lethargy, weakness, tremors, bloody urine and changes in thirst and urination in cats and dogs. Fortunately, shamrock tastes bitter so is rarely consumed in quantities large enough to cause any serious damage.

- **Star fruit** (*Averrhoa carambola*) Due to the oxalate salts in these fruits the signs of poisoning are the same as for shamrock above except star fruit are not bitter so may be more likely to be consumed.
- **Tobacco** (*Nicotiana tabacum*) Ingestion of nicotine from the plant, cigarettes or patches can lead to vomiting, tremors, collapse and death in cats and dogs.
- **Umbrella tree** (*Brassaia actinophylla, Schefflera arboricola*): Chewing or biting into this plant releases the crystals which penetrate tissue, resulting in injury. When dogs or cats ingest calcium oxalate-containing plants, signs may be seen immediately and include pawing at the face (oral pain), drooling, foaming and vomiting. Moderate to severe swelling of the lips, tongue, oral cavity and upper airway may also be seen, making it difficult to breathe or swallow.

More information about each plant, nutrient, health issue and other hazards to human health can be found in the 1130 pages of *Nature Cures – the A to Z of Ailments and Natural Foods* and the related website www.naturecures.co.uk.

Index

alfalfa, 24
allicin, 42
aloe vera, 98
amaryllis, 103
antioxidants, 20
ants, 12
aphids, 12
apples, 81
artichoke, 24
ash (burnt wood), 93
ashitaba, 25
asparagus, 26
assassin bugs, 14
aubergine, 27
autumn crocus, 104
avocado, 82, 104
azalea, 104
bay leaves, 104
basil, 56
beans, 28
beetroot, 30
bell peppers, 31
berries, 83
black fly, 12
bluebell, 105
bone meal, 95
borage, 58
brassicas, 10, 32
burdock, 58
cannabis, 106
carrots, 33
castor beans, 107
celery, 34
chamomile, 59
cherries, 84, 105
chicken pellets, 95
chicory, 60
chilli peppers, 34
chives, 61, 105
citrus fruit, 85
comfrey, 62, 95
compost, 95
coriander, 63
courgettes, 36
cucumber, 38
cyclamen, 105
damsel bug, 14
dandelion, 64
dill, 65
dragonfly, 14
dragon tree, 106
echinacea, 66
English ivy, 106
fennel, 66
fenugreek, 39
figs, 86
fish meal, 95
flowers, 90
foxgloves, 106
free radicals, 20
fruit, 81
fruit seeds/pips, 106
gall midge, 14
garlic, 40
ginger, 68
grapes, 88, 106
green fly, 12
heart leaf
    philodendron, 106

herbs, 55
hoverfly, 14
hops, 107
Japanese pieris, 107
Japanese yes, 107
jimson weed, 107
kalanchoe, 107
kelp, 96
kiwi fruit, 89
lacewing, 15
ladybird, 15
laurel, 104
lemons, 85
lemon balm, 70
lemongrass, 71
lemon thyme, 80
lily, 107
lily of the valley, 107
limes, 86
longhorn beetle, 15
manure, 96
marigold, 91
marjoram, 72
milk thistle, 72
mint, 73
mushrooms, 107
nasturtium, 91
nettles, 73

okra, 41
oleander, 107
onion, 42
oranges, 86
oregano, 75
parsley, 76
parsnips, 43
pears, 90
peppermint, 77
pirate bug, 15
poisonous plants, 103
potatoes, 44, 108
pothos, 108
praying mantis, 15
pumpkin, 45
radish, 46
rhubarb, 108
rosemary, 78
sage, 79
sago palm plant, 108
seaweed, 96
shamrock, 108
slugs, 17
snails, 17
soldier beetle, 15
spider mites, 19
spinach, 47
spring onions, 48

sprouting, 99-102
star fruit, 109
stinging nettles, 16
stink bug, 15
sunflowers, 92
swede, 48
sweet corn, 49
sweet potato, 50
swiss chard, 53
tarragon, 80
tangerines, 86
thyme, 80
tobacco, 109
tomatoes, 54
turnips, 55
umbrella tree, 109
vegetables, 23
wasps, 14, 15
water, 97
white fly, 12

About the Author

Nat Hawes SNHS Dip (Advanced Nutrition and Sports Nutrition) runs a successful Nutritional Therapy Clinic in London, England, where she deals with patients suffering from injury, surgery and infections, as well as from allergies, chronic fatigue, diabetes, digestive disorders, infertility, insomnia, obesity, pain and inflammation, mental health issues. She has spent 15 years researching and compiling her internationally popular website which brings together both the health problems that can be helped by nutritional interventions, and the healing properties of natural foods.

She can be contacted via www.naturecures.co.uk, health@naturecures.co.uk or the Nature Cures Nutritional Therapy Clinic (tel: +44(0)7783 940 999).